Plyometric

ANATOMY

Derek Hansen

Steve Kennelly

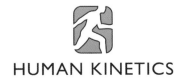

HUMAN KINETICS

Library of Congress Cataloging-in-Publication Data

Names: Hansen, Derek, 1969- author. | Kennelly, Steve, author.
Title: Plyometric anatomy / Derek Hansen, Steve Kennelly.
Description: Champaign, IL : Human Kinetics, [2017] | Includes
  bibliographical references and index.
Identifiers: LCCN 2017011257 (print) | LCCN 2017008863 (ebook) | ISBN
  9781492533498 (print) | ISBN 9781492535591 (ebook)
Subjects: LCSH: Physical fitness--Health aspects. | Exercise--Physiological
  aspects.
Classification: LCC RA781 .H343 2017 (ebook) | LCC RA781 (print) | DDC
  613.7--dc23
LC record available at https://lccn.loc.gov/2017011257

ISBN: 978-1-4925-3349-8 (print)

This publication is written and published to provide accurate and authoritative information relevant to the subject matter presented. It is published and sold with the understanding that the author and publisher are not engaged in rendering legal, medical, or other professional services by reason of their authorship or publication of this work. If medical or other expert assistance is required, the services of a competent professional person should be sought.

Acquisitions Editor: Jeff Mathis; **Senior Developmental Editor:** Cynthia McEntire; **Managing Editor:** Caitlin Husted; **Copyeditor:** Jan Feeney; **Permissions Manager:** Martha Gullo; **Graphic Designers:** Keri Evans and Denise Lowry; **Cover Designer**: Keri Evans; **Visual Production Assistant:** Joyce Brumfield; **Senior Art Manager:** Kelly Hendren; **Cover and Interior Illustrations:** © Human Kinetics; **Printer:** Versa Press

We thank Simon Fraser University in Burnaby, British Columbia, Canada, for assistance in providing the location for the photo shoot for this book.

Human Kinetics books are available at special discounts for bulk purchase. Special editions or book excerpts can also be created to specification. For details, contact the Special Sales Manager at Human Kinetics.

Printed in the United States of America   10 9 8 7 6 5 4 3 2 1

The paper in this book is certified under a sustainable forestry program.

Human Kinetics
Website: www.HumanKinetics.com

United States: Human Kinetics, P.O. Box 5076, Champaign, IL 61825-5076
800-747-4457
e-mail: info@hkusa.com

Canada: Human Kinetics, 475 Devonshire Road Unit 100, Windsor, ON N8Y 2L5
800-465-7301 (in Canada only)
e-mail: info@hkcanada.com

Europe: Human Kinetics, 107 Bradford Road, Stanningley, Leeds LS28 6AT, United Kingdom
+44 (0) 113 255 5665
e-mail: hk@hkeurope.com

For information about Human Kinetics' coverage in other areas of the world, please visit our website: www.HumanKinetics.com

E6832

To my unconditionally loving family for their endless support and patience. My wife, Carolyn, and my children, Callum, Bridgette, and Hannah, have always been there for me and provide me with the motivation to find better ways of helping people. I also want to thank my parents, Clarence and Carole, for urging me to follow my passions and always put forward my best effort. Finally, I would not be in a position to share my knowledge without the guidance of my mentors, including Al Vermeil, Rob Panariello, Donald Chu, Al Miller, Joseph Horrigan, and Charlie Francis.

Derek Hansen

To my wife Rita, and our children Ryan, Lia, and Mary. Thanks for your never ending love and support and for creating balance in our lives.

Steve Kennelly

CONTENTS

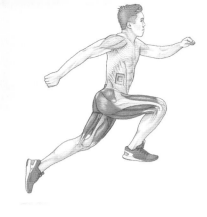

INTRODUCTION

The current emphasis on sport science and technology in all areas of human performance has encouraged athletes, coaches, and sport medicine professionals to seek out the most effective ways to train and closely monitor athletic improvement daily. Athletes not only desire to be consistently faster, stronger, and more powerful but also more resistant to injury. Staying resilient and healthy is as important to athletes as performing at a high level, because missed training sessions and competitions only make it more difficult to progress and maintain a high level of output. Thus, you need to take special care when selecting, arranging, and integrating training elements to elicit the desired responses and adaptations. Improving performance is not so much about finding the magic bullet of training but rather about developing a comprehensive approach composed of precise exercises dispensed at the most appropriate times of the training program.

Some of the most effective exercises for improving strength, power, and speed involve little to no equipment. While the sport training and fitness industries are inundated with all types of resistance training machines and speed training devices, the combination of gravity and the human body is all that is required. Over half a century ago, coaches and sport scientists developed an approach to training that took advantage of a system of explosive athletic movements to improve the force production qualities of the human body. This system of training is now commonly referred to as plyometrics. The term *plyometrics*—originally coined by U.S. runner and coach Fred Wilt in 1975—is derived from the Greek prefix *plio* meaning "more" or "longer" and the suffix "metric" meaning "to measure." While the literal translation of the word *plyometric* does not provide much information about the details of the system, it does imply a precise anatomical approach to exercise.

In its truest form, a plyometric exercise makes use of the body's natural response to the rapid lengthening of muscle. This response has also been referred to as the stretch-shortening cycle or myotatic reflex. Research has shown that a muscle stretched rapidly before a contraction will contract and shorten more forcefully and rapidly, creating positive adaptations for strength, power, and speed (Komi 1984; De Villarreal, Requena, and Newton 2010). For example, a basketball player preparing to grab a rebound will gather and lower his center of gravity before forcefully jumping up and securing the ball (figure 1). Similarly, a volleyball player will drop rapidly into a deep knee bend before jumping up to block an opposing player's spike attempt. It is a natural human response to load up or gather before an explosive movement. In golf, a back swing actively stretches the key muscles required for the powerful, high-velocity forward movement of the club. A baseball pitcher will wind up before delivering a high-speed pitch over home plate. You witness the benefits of plyometric activity in every sporting event. In some cases, athletes learn to resist resorting

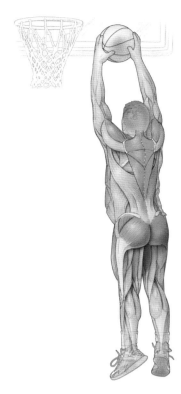

FIGURE 1   Basketball player securing a rebound after a power gather and jump.

to using the stretch-shortening cycle in order to save time, as in starting from blocks in both track sprinting and swimming competitions. In boxing and other combative sports, loading up for a punch can give the opponent time to prepare for an assault.

The term *plyometric* has been actively used since the 1960s to describe a system of exercises that improve performance. In many instances, plyometrics have been purported to be the invention of Eastern European nations, including Russia. While Russian coaches and sport scientists documented their use of plyometric exercises in training athletes, such exercises have likely been used for centuries by athletes competing in sporting activities requiring sprinting and jumping. By their nature, track and field events involve the specific involvement of the stretch-shortening cycle. Running and in particular sprinting (figure 2) can be considered the purest form of plyometric activity with each ground contact involving the stretching and contraction of muscles in the feet, lower leg, thigh, and hip, all occurring at a very high speed and over a very short time. The jumping events in track and field involve a gather step or penultimate stride that also loads the muscles and tendons and sets up an explosive jump for height or distance. The throwing events such as javelin, discus, and shot put also involve a combination of plyometric actions throughout the body to propel an implement over long distances.

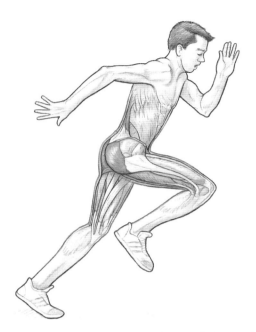

FIGURE 2   Fast running is one of the purest forms of plyometric activity.

Because plyometric actions are actively required in numerous track and field events, it makes sense that athletes and coaches would incorporate these activities into their training regimens (Bompa 1993). Sprinters would sprint over various distances, jumpers performed jumping activities, and throwers would throw their implements. Through repetition of these exercises in training, athletes would ultimately improve their performances. As the connection was made between these plyometric activities and enhanced performance, coaches began developing a systematic approach to incorporating these exercises into training programs, particularly during off-season training when inclement weather forced them indoors and coaches had to be creative with workouts. It was not until the late 1960s that sport scientists started to look closer at the benefits of plyometric exercise and investigate optimal protocols for enhancing athletic performance.

Yuri Verkhoshansky was one of the first to undertake studies of various methods of plyometric jumps to determine optimal methods of training. Verkhoshansky's (1973) shock method of training involved jumping from a height and rebounding to improve jumping strength and simulate the function required for explosive athletic movements. He found that completed depth jumps from a relatively significant height for 40 repetitions for two training sessions per week was effective in building dynamic strength and speed abilities. Others began to recognize the value in quantifying the precise implementation of plyometric jumps and developed a comprehensive approach to integrating these exercises with an overall training plan. Dr. Donald Chu (1984), who has written numerous articles and books on the subject, identified plyometric training as a method of bridging the gap between power and speed. He also indicated that while the exercises can provide significant benefits, the system of plyometric training is most important in providing sustainable improvements.

When plyometric training was introduced to the United States in the early 1970s, it was presented as a revolutionary training phenomenon (Holcomb, Kleiner, and Chu 1998). In the present sporting world, plyometric exercises are a staple of explosive power training for athletes of all ages and abilities. These exercises are widely accepted by training professionals as a means of improving strength, power, and speed in all athletes (Simenz, Dugan, and Ebben 2005; Ebben, Carroll, and Simenz 2004; Ebben, Hintz, and Simenz 2005). In addition, more recent research has indicated that plyometric training has significant benefits for endurance athletes by improving the economy of movement over longer durations (Spurrs, Murphy, and Watsford 2003; Saunders, Telford, and Pyne 2006).

In *Plyometric Anatomy*, we provide an array of plyometric exercises for enhanced athletic performance and a precise means of targeting the specific muscles and connective tissues involved in explosive movements in all sports. The visual presentation of these exercises and associated anatomy also provides greater insight on avoiding overuse conditions and preventing injuries. Although many plyometric exercises rely on the same muscles, tendons, and ligaments for the delivery of force and transfer of power, subtle differences in biomechanics and technical execution can mean the difference between a profound training effect and a potential injury.

This book utilizes the use of color coding the primary and secondary muscles in specific exercises (as seen in the key). The darker-colored muscles are the primary muscles used while the lighter-colored muscles are the secondary muscles used in the exercise.

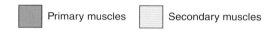

Plyometric Anatomy examines the science and physiology behind plyometric training and identifies both foundational and advanced exercises. Exercises are presented in a logical progression, starting with basic movements and advancing to more intense and complex movements. Exercises for upper- and lower-body training are presented as well as specific movements for core development. For advanced athletes who have a substantial base of training, we provide combination exercises that simulate complex sport-specific movements. As Yuri Verkhoshansky (1969) suggested, it is imperative to model strength and power training as closely as possible to the function that is to be improved. This book also presents key measures for prevention and rehabilitation of injuries related to use and management of plyometric training. The visual nature of this training resource makes it a valuable tool in the pursuit of enhanced performance and a healthy career in all sports.

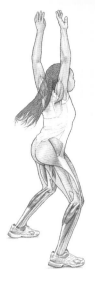

PHYSIOLOGICAL MECHANISM OF PLYOMETRICS

In many ways, the use of plyometric exercises was borne out of the need to manage the force of gravity, whether for reasons of survival in ancient times or, more recently, in the pursuit of sporting excellence. Gathering for a jump, sprint, or throw reflects an athlete's natural tendency to develop a strategy to overcome gravity or inertia of an object or the athlete's own body in an effort to produce a more forceful effort. Although it may appear to be a simple strategy, the physiological mechanisms involved in the execution of plyometric movements are quite advanced and involve a series of coordinated and synergistic muscular actions for maximal results. To best explain the physiological mechanisms and anatomical structures behind plyometrics, it is necessary to understand the key muscular actions and anatomy involved in these exercises.

MUSCULAR ACTIONS IN PLYOMETRICS

One of the most common examples of a plyometric action is the stride cycle of a running athlete. When an athlete lands a stride, the muscles of the involved leg lengthen rapidly due to the force of the athlete's body being drawn to the ground by gravity. Eccentric muscle actions throughout the hip and leg prevent the athlete from collapsing by slowly resisting the lengthening of these muscles. In addition to preventing an excessive drop in the body's center of mass, eccentric muscular actions help dampen the impact of landing. Eccentric muscle contractions throughout the lower extremities, hips, and torso act collectively as the body's shock absorbers, minimizing excessive forces on connective tissues and skeletal structures. The forces experienced by the muscles during eccentric muscular contractions can be greater than 40 percent of those of other muscular actions, as demonstrated by the magnitude of force felt on the landings of a stride or jump (Chu and Myer 2013). Without these shock absorbers, an athlete's body would undergo a good deal of punishment on every landing of a jump or stride, ultimately resulting in serious injury.

Once the muscles decelerate and stop the downward path of the body on ground contact of a running stride, for a brief period the muscles do not lengthen or shorten. The joints of the lower body—such as the knee and ankle—are fixed during this short time, with no flexion or extension occurring. When the muscles are in a static state of constant tension with no movement occurring, an isometric muscle contraction is taking place. In the case of the running stride and similar plyometric activities, isometric muscle contractions are of very short duration and precede the reversal of muscular action from lengthening to shortening. A runner lands on the ground with a stride, absorbs the force of the landing, and then ultimately pushes up and forward to enter the flight phase of the stride cycle. This isometric action, also referred to as the coupling phase, is critical to producing the power required for forceful muscular contractions in plyometric activities.

Once the action of muscle lengthening is slowed, stopped, and reversed, the shortening of muscle required for creating powerful movements is referred to as a concentric muscular contraction. Concentric muscle actions are the product of plyometric activities and, in the case of a running stride cycle, result in the push-off phase of the stride that vaults an athlete into the flight phase. The concentric muscle action can be seen when a high jumper takes off or a basketball player leaps toward the hoop on a layup. A concentric muscle action also occurs after a baseball pitcher winds up and begins the forward delivery of a throw toward home plate. In many ways, the concentric action is what typically receives the most attention in sporting performances: the takeoff for a jump, the delivery of a throw, or the stealth execution of a knockout punch. However, great performances are the product of the entire array of muscle actions, perfectly timed and efficiently executed. Figure 1.1 identifies all muscle actions taking place throughout the running stride cycle.

A similar combination of eccentric, isometric, and concentric muscle actions takes place in numerous movements in various sports. These actions have also been identified as the loading, coupling, and unloading phases, respectively.

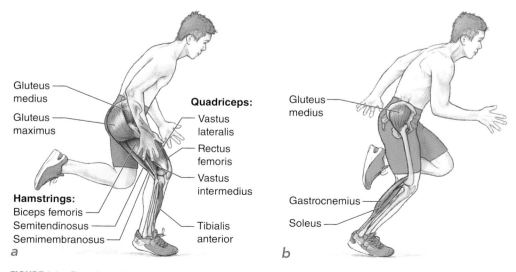

FIGURE 1.1 Running stride cycle.

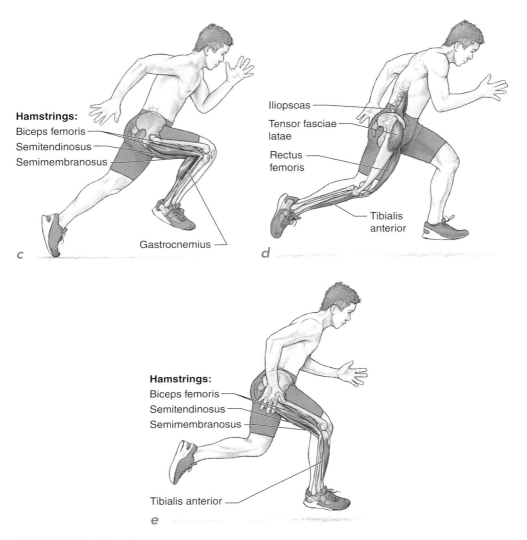

FIGURE 1.1 *(continued)*

It is important for coaches and athletes to understand these components of a plyometric activity in order to best use individual exercises to enhance various aspects of athleticism. In many cases, the joint angles achieved and the time spent in these various muscle actions determine which exercises to choose for a particular phase of a training program. A skilled coach will provide an optimal progression of exercises that safely enhance performance from phase to phase to ensure an athlete peaks at the right time.

STRETCH-SHORTENING CYCLE

The combination of muscle actions, neural involvement, and connective tissue elasticity that facilitate an effective plyometric action can be explained more readily through a discussion of the stretch-shortening cycle (SSC). When the combination of muscle and tendon are rapidly stretched, as is the case in a fast eccentric movement, the nervous system responds by recruiting a larger proportion of muscle fiber to produce greater force in an effort to reverse the direction of movement (Komi 1984). The muscle-tendon complex senses the rapid lengthening via the muscle spindle fibers that are specific sensory organs located within the muscle, as illustrated in figure 1.2. The muscle spindle fibers monitor the lengthening of muscle as well as the velocity of lengthening, responding with a forceful concentric contraction of muscle. These built-in responses to the rapid lengthening of muscle ensure that athletes do not need to overtly think about powerfully contracting their muscles for an explosive effort. The collective mechanisms involved in the stretch-shortening cycle have been identified as the stretch reflex, tendon elasticity, preactivation, and potentiation (Fukutani, Kurihara, and Isaka 2015). There has been much discussion, but little agreement, on the relative contributions of these various mechanisms to the stretch-shortening cycle (Komi 2000).

The stretch reflex, also referred to as the myotatic reflex, is a key mechanism for the stretch-shortening cycle and production of force in a plyometric exercise. While a proportion of force in a plyometric movement is from the basic elastic energy released from the elastic qualities of both muscles and tendons, similar to an elastic band, a significant contribution of force comes from the rapid recruitment of muscle fiber elicited by the stretch reflex. In fact, research has demonstrated that the rapid lengthening of muscle results in the selective activation of fast-twitch muscle fibers and the deactivation of slow-twitch muscle fibers (Nardone and Schieppati 1988). The stretch reflex is demonstrated every day in a physician's office when reflex testing is carried out with the use of a rubber mallet. A quick tap of the patellar tendon typically elicits a shortening of the quadriceps muscles and the extension of the knee joint in a healthy person. Signals from the muscle spindle fibers to the spinal cord trigger a rapid response, at a velocity of approximately 100 meters per second, to recruit the

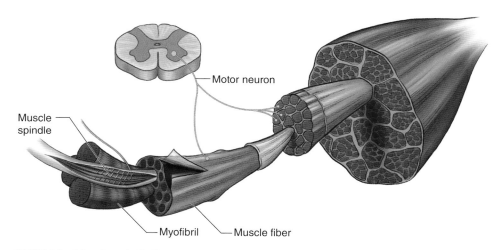

FIGURE 1.2   Muscle spindle fiber in the muscle belly.

quadriceps muscle (Radcliffe and Farentinos 1985). The primary purpose of the stretch reflex is to monitor the magnitude of muscle stretch as a safety precaution to prevent excessive stretching and damage to the muscle. By recruiting a large proportion of muscle fiber in any given muscle in a very short time, this automatic response ensures that the muscle lengthens only to a safe degree before engaging in shortening. While it may be considered an automatically regulated safety measure, coaches and sport scientists have found it advantageous to safely train this response for the purpose of enhanced performance.

Sport science professionals often refer to the amortization phase, or transition phase, to describe the start of the eccentric contraction all the way through to the beginning of the concentric contraction in a plyometric movement. The amortization phase is the period in which an athlete prepares for an explosive movement such as a jump. For a long jumper, the amortization phase includes the beginning of touchdown on the takeoff board through the point of the beginning of the takeoff movement as the athlete's center of mass passes over the foot. For athletes who jump for height or distance, a long amortization phase is undesirable because it results in a significant loss of power. Not only does a long amortization phase squander any elastic contribution to the jump, but it also limits the activation potential of the stretch reflex and the resulting force of concentric contraction. Thus, it is in the best interests of athletes to shorten the duration of the amortization phase when executing a powerful plyometric action (Wilson, Elliott, and Wood 1991). The magnitude of the force applied to the amortization phase will determine the resulting force of contraction for the concentric portion of the muscle action, particularly in a well-trained athlete.

PROPERTIES OF MUSCLE AND TENDON

The muscle spindle fibers are the primary sensory mechanism for triggering a powerful concentric contraction in a plyometric movement. Another sensory organ in the muscle-tendon unit is the Golgi tendon organ (figure 1.3). This particular stretch receptor is located in the tendons and, when stretched forcefully, transmits signals to the spinal cord to create an inhibitory response to a contracted muscle. In this way, the action of the Golgi tendon organ has been portrayed as a protective mechanism to prevent the muscle from excessive tension and potential injury. This reflex mechanism is demonstrated when a person jumps from an extreme height and collapses to the ground, sometimes rolling out of the landing to dissipate forces and avoid injury. It is important to recognize that both of these sensory organs may come into play when planning and implementing a plyometric exercise program, particularly when identifying optimal jump heights. A jump from a box at a moderate height may produce enough force to create an eccentric stretch that activates the muscle spindles for a powerful concentric response. However, a jump from an excessively high box may stretch a tendon rapidly and invoke an inhibitory response from Golgi tendon organs, ultimately shutting down a concentric contraction.

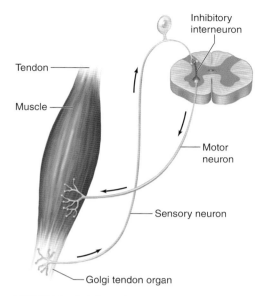

Inhibitory interneuron

Tendon

Muscle

Motor neuron

Sensory neuron

Golgi tendon organ

FIGURE 1.3   Golgi tendon organ.

While the sensory mechanisms required for an explosive muscular response are critical elements in plyometrics, the contractile components of muscle play a significant role in the creation of movement. The basic force-generating elements of muscle are the actin and myosin myofilaments formed from individual actin and myosin molecules. These myofilaments collectively make up the myofibrils in individual muscle fibers. These muscle fibers form larger bundles of the muscle fasciculi that combine to make up the skeletal muscles that create human movement. In a contracting muscle, movement is initiated when the actin and myosin filaments form cross-bridges and slide past one another. The sliding action occurs through a cyclic attachment and detachment of myosin on the actin filaments (Spudich 2001). When a muscle is stretched while activated, the isometric force achieved after the stretch is higher than that produced during normal isometric contractions at the same length (Abbott and Aubert 1952; Rassier et al. 2003). It has been suggested that force enhancement and increased stiffness are associated with cross-bridge mechanics: The proportion of cross-bridges after a stretch is higher than that associated with an isometric contraction (Herzog and Leonard 2000).

Other elements that contribute to the explosive-performance properties of muscle are known as the series elastic components. In series elastic components, muscle fibers, including the cross-bridging elements of actin and myosin myofilaments, are connected in line with elastic structures such as tendons. The elongation of these series elastic components during muscle contractions produces potential energy similar to that of a loaded spring or a stretched rubber band (Hill 1950). As mentioned previously, if the amortization phase of a plyometric movement is too long, the potential energy stored in the elasticity of muscles will dissipate and the benefits of eccentric loading are lost, primarily in the form of heat energy (Cavagna 1977). The rate of loading has been found to be of more consequence than the length or magnitude of stretch in a muscle-tendon complex (Bosco and Komi 1979). An important consideration in any plyometric exercise is to ensure that the loading phase and prestretch of the series elastic components are quick, resulting in a more explosive and elastic movement.

CENTRAL NERVOUS SYSTEM

While the anatomical components are critical for the structural and mechanical execution of the muscular contractions involved in plyometric exercises, the neurological energy and "software" required to power the "hardware" are equally important. Because explosive movements require maximal recruitment of available muscle fiber, significant neural involvement is imperative. Regardless of the size of a muscle, if the appropriate signals are not being sent from the brain and spinal cord (the central nervous system), a maximal effort will not be realized for explosive movements. The involvement of the nervous system in the development of strength, power, and speed is demonstrated by the cross-education effect of training, particularly in cases when one limb is recovering from injury. When the muscles of the uninjured limb are subjected to a voluntary strength training program, the same muscles of the opposite untrained limb have a 10 to 15 percent increase in strength over the same period (Enoka 1997). While many athletes believe that building big, strong muscles is the key to improving strength, power, and speed, the contributions of neuromuscular adaptations must not be overlooked when developing an optimal plyometric training program.

As with any movement that involves speed, power, or maximum strength, adequate recovery times between bouts of intense jumps or throws are required in order to allow for reproduction of maximal performance in both training and competition. Athletes who are fully recovered and who display an appropriate state of readiness will always benefit from plyometric training more than athletes who are fatigued. Research shows that as much as 5 minutes of recovery time after a bout of fatiguing stretch-shortening cycle training may be required for achieving equal or superior subsequent performances (Comyns, Harrison, and Hennessy 2011). It is not surprising that many sport scientists are now implementing drop jumps on force plates and contact mats as a means of measuring both central and peripheral fatigue in athletes and monitoring overall athlete recovery and readiness with the use of the stretch-shortening cycle.

The next few chapters identify primary concepts for implementing a proper progression of loading using various exercises and types of equipment. You will also find key foundational exercises that you should perform before embarking on a comprehensive strength, power, and speed training program. These foundational exercises are the building blocks for many more advanced and complex exercises used in the pursuit of high performance. All exercises are presented with detailed illustrations identifying key anatomical structures involved in the execution of these explosive movements. Awareness of the specific muscles and connective tissues involved in a plyometric program can provide greater insights into not only the technical execution of these exercises but also the movements and protocols required for warming up, cooling down, and facilitating recovery.

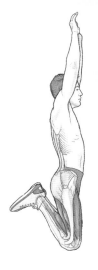

TRAINING PROGRESSIONS, SURFACES, AND EQUIPMENT

Embarking on a plyometric training program can be an elaborate task. A significant amount of planning and preparation will likely be required for properly integrating appropriate plyometric routines into an overall training program. Because of the explosive and technical nature of plyometric activities, a gradual progression of exercises and techniques is needed for maximizing both efficiency and safety. While plyometric training has been proven effective in improving strength, power, and speed, you must take special care to ensure appropriate preparation to implement the exercises effectively and with adequate recovery between individual sets and sessions. Exercise selection, work volume, training surface, and equipment selection are all important considerations before starting a plyometric program.

PRELIMINARY STEPS

Some suggest that an athlete must be able to squat a specific amount of weight before participating in a plyometric training program. A commonly cited prerequisite for explosive jumps is 1.5 times an athlete's body weight for a back squat. The logic behind this assertion is that a minimum level of strength is required for safely handling the forces experienced in dynamic plyometric activities. Conventional wisdom dictates that the muscles and tendons must have a base of strength to handle the demands of explosive activities. While it is convenient to put a specific number on the absolute strength required for plyometric activity, there are many ways to prepare for the demands of such a program. In fact, many of the activities performed by children as a part of their regular play routines can be considered preparatory movements. The running, skipping, and jumping observed in a playground environment can all be considered early introductions to plyometric activities. In addition, many sport-specific movements are inherently plyometric, particularly in sports such as volleyball and basketball, and are performed every day throughout practices and games.

An easy way to introduce plyometric activities—particularly for those who are new to the training method—is to be selective with the types of exercises implemented. In the preparatory phases of a plyometric program, exercises that limit landing and eccentric stresses are preferred. Another consideration is the surface used for plyometric activities. Softer surfaces, although not optimal for activation of the stretch reflex, are a good place to start to minimize impact stresses. As the training program progresses and strength improves, incorporate harder surfaces and more dynamic jumps into the overall program to activate the stretch reflex and simulate the specifics of the sport surface of competition. A proper progression of exercises, surfaces, and equipment improves performance efficiently and maximizes safety.

In all cases when intense exercise is to be performed, you should undergo a comprehensive medical examination before the start of the program. An understanding of injury history and any preexisting medical conditions will help to determine appropriate exercises and rates of progression. For example, if you have a history of knee or low back pain, you may require lower volumes of work and a more gradual progression of loading to minimize the incidence of pain or further injury.

EXERCISE PROGRESSIONS

Using the correct exercises at the appropriate time in a training program is key to ensuring enough stimulation for a positive adaptation but without creating excessive stress that can lead to injury. For a program that is ultimately preparing for explosive plyometric jumps, take care to introduce exercises that are not too complex or stressful. At the same time, the initial steps of a plyometric program should be stressful enough to lead to a progression to the next level.

One of the most basic exercises is a jump onto a box or platform to train concentric jumping abilities. Jumping onto a box provides the benefit of training explosive extension at the hip, knee, and ankle (also known as triple extension) without the impact of a stressful landing. Ideally, the box height will be just below the height of the apex of the jump so you are able to complete the jump safely but also land just after you begin to descend.

Initially, you can jump onto a box or platform at a static start position from various squat depths as illustrated in figure 2.1. You can perform quicker jumps to a low- or moderate-height box with a small degree of knee flexion at the start. You can do more powerful jumps to a higher box from a deeper knee bend. In both cases, the emphasis is on a quick concentric motion that does not require you to gather for the movement.

Once you have demonstrated competence in the static-start box jump, move to countermovement jumps. Initiating a strong downward countermovement gives you access to the benefits of the stretch-shortening cycle to produce greater force for the upward jump. The landing on top of the box is the same as for a static-start jump—land softly after the apex of the jump.

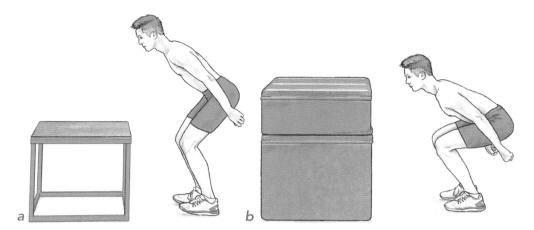

FIGURE 2.1   Static start positions for jumps onto a box: *(a)* little knee flexion; *(b)* deeper knee bend.

Other jumping methods that can be used early in a training program are basic jumps in place in a swimming pool. The water provides resistance for the concentric portion of a jump and a significant amount of unloading for the landing phase due to buoyancy in the water. Chest-deep water is a perfect environment for introducing jumps in place that develop strength and power. Perform basic squat jumps initially, one repetition at a time, to work on posture, jumping technique, and landing strategy. As you progress over several sessions, add rebounding jumps that introduce low to moderate loading of plyometric qualities. The pool environment allows progress into jumps over distance as well; the water provides external resistance to movement while challenging balance on landings. The forgiving nature of the pool environment demonstrates how it can be useful for incorporating and reintroducing plyometrics in the context of rehabilitation and return-to-competition training.

As strength and power improve through concentric jumps and moderate-load landings, exercises gradually move into more demanding landing scenarios. Jumps in place are a good means of continuing to develop concentric power while incorporating technical work on landing mechanics. While many athletes know how to jump and take off, other athletes may require more work on the technical aspects of landing safely. A simple squat jump in place can be used to train all aspects of the jumping motion. On landing, learn to properly absorb the forces of a landing through multiple joints and muscle groups, decelerating the body appropriately. As you demonstrate good landing mechanics, progress to multiple jumps in place, such as multiple squat jumps. Initially, these jumps do not need to be high; simply focus on absorbing force and reversing the body's direction from descending to ascending. These low-amplitude jumps not only provide appropriate training stress but also give you time to develop proper technique and timing with lower intensity. As training progresses, jumps in place can become more aggressive, with greater height and shorter ground contact time.

Gradually, low-amplitude jumps in place progress to jumps over distance, adding a horizontal component to the movement. Horizontal travel adds complexity to the movement and stresses the body in a new way to combat the body's gradual adaptation. As with jumps in place, you can introduce lower-amplitude jumps over distance initially, with greater heights and distances for individual jumps improving from week to week. You can perform a low-height pogo jump in place over a 5- to 10-meter distance with low, short jumps of no more than 30 centimeters per jump in the initial phases of a horizontal progression. These jumps can gradually increase to 50-centimeter lengths and also increase in height as you adapt to both the horizontal and vertical forces.

Another variable managed through the implementation of plyometric progressions is the use of two legs versus one leg for jumping movements. It is generally accepted that double-leg movements are relatively less stressful and less complex than single-leg movements. Jumps with a single leg can provide a greater proprioceptive challenge, necessitating stable landings and additional hip and knee control. Single-leg jumps can be used to simulate single-leg takeoffs in jumping sports as well as prepare the body for cutting movements used in various sports and agility training. Thus introduce double-leg jumps initially in a training program and then integrate single-leg movements gradually as strength, stability, and technical competence increase. In many ways, the transition from double-leg to single-leg exercises can be seen as a trend from general work to more specific work in a training program.

As you progress to maximal-effort jumps over distance, extend the distances to provide additional load. Initially, jumps may be over 10 meters, with five to seven jumps constituting a single set. Sets may be expanded to 20 to 30 meters and include improvements in both vertical height and horizontal velocity. It is important to progress carefully when adding both height and distance to your jumps over multiple repetitions and sets because the overall loading stresses can rapidly accumulate to a point where fatigue is excessive and the risk of injury significantly increases.

Add vertical barriers in the form of hurdles to provide tangible goals of height for multiple jumps. Select hurdle heights that encourage you to jump maximally, but avoid excessive heights that increase the risk of tripping and falling. Athletes often enjoy the feeling of jumping over a barrier as part of a plyometric routine to give them a sense of achievement and an indication of jump height. Lower hurdles can be advantageous for large groups of athletes with varying jumping abilities. Less explosive athletes can still jump over lower hurdles safely, while more explosive athletes can simply jump higher over the lower hurdles and still accomplish an effective workout session.

Depth jumps specifically target the stretch-shortening cycle with the use of precise box heights. In a depth jump, you step off a low- to moderate-height box, descend to the floor, then perform a maximal reactive jump back into the air. The exercise can be set up so that you jump onto a higher box or over a relatively high hurdle after jumping back into the air. Each repetition is carefully set up to ensure that the drop is consistently executed and a relatively short ground-contact time is achieved on the reactive jump. A depth-jump session can be a stressful workout because of the magnitude of load experienced at ground contact, particularly if a taller box is used. In most cases, athletes perform two-foot jumps because of the impact stress. You can perform single-leg depth jumps, but drop heights must be relatively low so you maintain short ground-contact time and minimize the risk of injury. In a plyometric jump progression, you may use depth jumps in the latter stages of a preparatory phase after you have accumulated a significant amount of strength through other types of jumps and plyometric exercises as well as strength and power contributions from conventional weight training.

As a further step in the progression, you can perform combinations of hurdle and box jumps in series to create a challenging but enjoyable experience. Drop off a box and then jump over hurdles or onto other boxes in an organized obstacle course of vertical barriers and platforms. It is important to have an appropriate combination of heights of boxes and hurdles to ensure that the equipment elicits maximal output on every jump while not overloading or exhausting you. As with any plyometric exercise routine, the intent is not to burden you with fatigue but to elicit the maximal stretch response from connective tissues. High-quality plyometric work results in positive adaptations for power and speed that enhance overall performance in your sport.

Figure 2.2 illustrates a conceptual approach to progressing into and through plyometric activities over the course of a training program. Early in the program, the intent is to introduce less stressful, less complex movements that provide foundational strength and coordination for subsequent exercises in the progression. The rate at which you can move through the progression depends on age, ability, experience, body weight, and existing strength level. For example, an athlete younger than 10 years may use only the first few stages of the plyometric progression spread over his entire training season. Simple box jumps and jumps in place provide adequate stimulus for improvements in strength and power while not risking injury. However, an older and more advanced athlete may move quickly through the entire progression, using different exercise types at the same time if she has experience with a comprehensive plyometric program

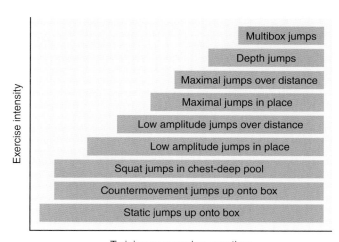

Training progression over time

FIGURE 2.2 Sample plyometric progression throughout a training season.

over several training seasons. A larger, heavier athlete may never progress up to hurdle jumps or depth jumps because of the risk of injury. Hence, a 350-pound American football lineman requires a significantly different plyometric progression than a 175-pound basketball point guard of the same age and level of development. General guidelines for implementing a safe and effective plyometric progression are useful when individualizing a training program.

While you will carry out most of these jumps in a linear fashion, you can introduce additional complexity by including rotational movements and lateral jumps. For box jumps with a static start or a countermovement, jump up and land with a 90-degree turn in either direction. You can also add rotational movements to jumps in place or over distance. Consider incorporation of rotational movements and lateral jumps advanced techniques that improve overall coordination and landing ability in a multidirectional fashion.

TRAINING SURFACES

The choice of training environment can have a significant impact on the effects of plyometric exercises for both training specificity and injury prevention. This is absolutely true of the choice of training surfaces for jumps and other explosive movements. The hardness of the ground can affect the amortization phase of a plyometric activity by either increasing or decreasing the ground-contact time.

A softer training surface typically results in a longer ground-contact time than a harder training surface. An extreme example of this concept is the effect of a trampoline on jumping. When a person lands on a trampoline, his body stiffens to take advantage of the elastic properties of the trampoline surface. Thus the body compensates for the softer landing surface by stiffening to elicit a desired response (bouncing up and down on the trampoline). On a harder training surface, the body does the opposite and softens connective tissues to provide a softer landing and a more appropriate elastic response. This muscle and tendon tuning effect has been demonstrated through research and allows the body to regulate ground reaction forces appropriately for both performance and safety.

Athletes who want to perform at the peak of their abilities in sprinting or jumping activities typically prefer to compete on harder surfaces to maximize the elastic potential of their bodies. However, it is advisable to train on slightly softer surfaces throughout the majority of the season to minimize soft-tissue injuries and maintain health during higher-volume preparatory periods.

These examples illustrate the importance of finding an appropriate balance of surface types throughout a training and competitive season. Following are specific examples of surface types that can be used throughout a training program to elicit specific training effects and minimize chronic and acute injury.

Sand

Athletes and coaches often use sand-based surfaces for jumping and running exercises in a preparatory phase of training to minimize impact stresses on the lower extremities. The displacement of loose sand on the landing of a jump can significantly dampen landing forces and reduce overall stresses on the muscles, tendons, and other connective tissues. As jumping and landing exercises are introduced in a training program, conducting plyometric activities on a beach surface or sand pit enables a greater number of repetitions, allowing you to acquire appropriate skills. Additionally, many sand-based exercises can be performed in bare feet, strengthening the numerous muscles of the feet on a softer, forgiving surface.

For concentric or plyometric activities, a sand-based surface creates a condition in which there is a reduced reliance on elastic properties of muscle and tendon because a longer concentric phase is incurred as the sand is displaced on a pushing stride or takeoff. While a sand-based environment can be helpful in introducing jump and landing mechanics, it is not recommended to spend too long training on this type of surface. Because it is more difficult to trigger a reflexive response on an extremely soft surface, the concern is that you could detrain the stretch reflex. The landing forces would be dissipated by the sand and not absorbed through the muscles and tendons of the lower extremities.

Grass

Natural grass is one of the best training surfaces. It is firm enough for the rapid production of force for running and jumping but also compliant enough to provide adequate cushioning on landings. Natural grass also has a relatively good combination of vertical and horizontal compliance on ground contact when landing a jump, running stride, or quick-deceleration step. This reduces the stresses on ligaments and tendons during explosive movements required for rapid acceleration or change of direction. These qualities make natural grass a good all-around surface for most, if not all, plyometric exercises throughout a training season. Note that grass surfaces vary in hardness depending on the local climate and frequency of irrigation. Drier conditions typically yield a harder grass surface, and you may need to take this into consideration when implementing plyometric activities.

Artificial Turf

Artificial turf surfaces can provide a good combination of firmness and shock absorption for athletic movements. In many cases, artificial surfaces also provide a greater degree of surface uniformity because natural surfaces can be uneven and riddled with divots and other irregularities. In wet conditions, artificial turf typically maintains its surface quality and firmness, while natural grass can become waterlogged and too soft for plyometric activities. In general, artificial turf surfaces can be harder than most natural grass surfaces, particularly if they are improperly maintained and not regularly groomed. Athletes can initiate a plyometric program on an artificial turf surface because it provides suitable cushioning for landings in most cases, in addition to a stable surface for dynamic movements. Harder artificial turf surfaces should be substituted with a softer grass surface, if possible, in the early stages of a plyometric progression. It is also important to recognize that artificial turf surfaces have a higher coefficient of friction (provide more grip) than a natural grass surface, and jumps and movements with greater horizontal force production can create more stresses on muscles, joints, and connective tissues. Lower volumes and intensities of these types of exercises may be introduced on artificial turf surfaces in a more gradual fashion. Considerations for footwear during training are also important: Use higher-traction footwear in the latter stages of the program to provide specificity without overloading.

Hardwood Court Floors

Hardwood surfaces are common for basketball, volleyball, and racket sports, including squash, racquetball, and badminton. In general, hardwood floors provide a firm but slightly dampened surface for sporting activities. As with all sport surfaces, there is some variability in hardness depending on the composition and construction of the flooring. Some may be very soft and compliant, while others may be very firm. More modern hardwood floors have been engineered to provide appropriate cushioning. Older floors may still be very stiff and less forgiving. Because choices to use indoor training activities are often dictated by weather and other seasonal factors, athletes may find themselves on hardwood court surfaces for the majority of their training. It is the responsibility of coaches and athletes to determine the condition of the training surface and make adjustments as necessary. This may mean starting the plyometric program on a softer outdoor training surface or, if no such option is available, modifying the program to incorporate less stressful movements in a more gradual fashion on a hardwood floor court surface.

Rubberized Tracks and Flooring

Synthetic track and sport surfaces are commonly used for sprint and plyometric training. The advantage of these types of surfaces is that they are very responsive for reactive jumping activities and other explosive movements. The downside of using these surfaces is that they can also be very hard, and extensive training on such surfaces can be stressful on the joints, muscles, and connective tissues. For track and field athletes who spend a good deal of their training on a synthetic track surface, use of a softer surface (grass, artificial turf) for the initial stages of plyometric training is a sound approach for staying healthy during the preparatory phases of a training program. Transitioning to a synthetic track surface for explosive and reactive jumps in the latter stages of a training program can be more easily accommodated because the athletes will be stronger and more resilient. The stiffer elastic surface of a track or rubberized floor can enhance the effect of a plyometric program, taking advantage of the stretch reflex for explosive and elastic movements. Athletes who compete on synthetic track surfaces should spend adequate time training on these surfaces to ensure that they are accustomed to the qualities and characteristics of the competition environment.

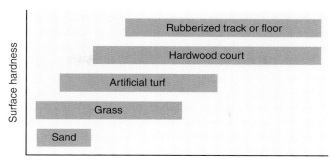

FIGURE 2.3 Plyometric-surface progression over a training program.

Figure 2.3 summarizes a progression of the use of various surfaces in a plyometric training program. A commonsense approach is to move from softer to harder surfaces over the duration of a training program to prevent excessive stress on the body too quickly. Ultimately, a training program should prepare you for the competitive environment. For example, soccer players train mostly on grass and turf, and beach volleyball players spend the majority of time on sandy beaches.

Take care to ensure that the specific demands of a sport are accommodated without spending excessive time on just one training surface. Varying the training surface has many benefits. Softer surfaces can dampen impact stresses and build strength qualities in muscles and connective tissues. Harder surfaces trigger an effective stretch–reflex response for explosive movements, providing neurological and elastic benefits that can transfer to other movements and surfaces. The right combination of surfaces depends on the sport, athlete, and many other circumstances such as weather, time of day, and fatigue. Make the best decision on training progression and surface choice.

FOOTWEAR

The choice of appropriate footwear for any training program can be critical in both performance and health. In running and jumping activities, the feet are the point of contact with the ground. Not only do the feet deliver the impacts that produce a stride, jump, or change of direction, but they also serve as sensory mechanisms that gather information on the quality of the surface. The feet indicate whether the ground is soft or hard, even or uneven, and "grippy" or slippery. Hence, the choice of footwear can be critical on many levels.

Sport shoes are, first and foremost, intended to protect the feet from damage and the wear and tear of daily sporting activities. Foot protection includes proper covering of the foot to avoid cuts and abrasions, adequate cushioning beneath the foot to absorb the shock of impacts, and appropriate support through the length of the shoe to brace the arch of the foot and prevent the foot from rolling laterally. While some athletes prefer to perform plyometric activities in bare feet, it is advisable to protect the feet with proper shoes for the majority of training sessions.

When training is limited to harder surfaces, the selection of footwear can be critical for reducing landing forces transferred to the body. An appropriately cushioned shoe can be used early in the training program and with harder surfaces for this reason. As strength develops, transition to a stiffer shoe that allows you to take advantage of the stretch reflex and elasticity stored in the connective tissues. You also may consider using a shoe with a thicker heel initially, providing less heel travel—and less posterior connective tissue stretch—on ground contact with the ball of the foot. The heel may contact the ground more with this type of shoe, but as strength improves, a shoe with a more even profile from heel to toe can be introduced. Figure 2.4 illustrates the difference in heel travel with a higher-heeled shoe and a more even-profile shoe.

As you progress from the early preparatory phases of plyometric training to more specific precompetitive phases, you may wish to carry out plyometric training in the shoes used for competition. In track and field, jumping and sprinting athletes may choose to participate in plyometrics with competition spikes in the lead-up to the competition phase. Track and field spikes provide significantly less cushioning and a flatter profile than regular running shoes, and training volumes must be adjusted accordingly to ensure volumes of ground contacts are kept to a minimum. A similar approach can be applied to cleats used in soccer, American football, baseball, and rugby, as well as court shoes used in racket sports, basketball, and volleyball.

Coaches can provide recommendations to athletes on the best shoe for various phases of training. While there is a push to make all training as specific as possible, it is always best to consider the advantages of varying footwear choices to achieve the best possible performance and health outcomes.

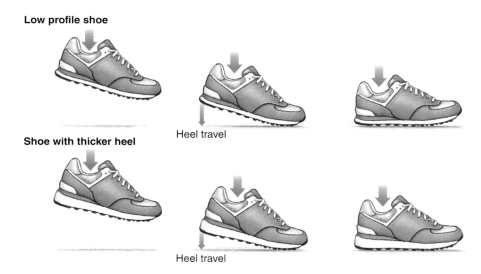

Low profile shoe

Heel travel

Shoe with thicker heel

Heel travel

FIGURE 2.4 Heel travel on ground contact with shoes of various heel thickness.

EQUIPMENT

While the progression of work with various exercises over various surfaces is critical in determining the effectiveness and safety of a plyometric program, the selection of equipment for plyometric activities can have a significant bearing on health and performance. Following are examples of equipment that can be considered for use in a plyometric training program.

Plyometric Boxes

The choice of plyometric boxes for jump training is often determined by financial means. Where boxes are not available, innovative coaches and athletes have implemented similar jumping routines using staircases and stadium bleachers for performing upward jumps in series. However, simple boxes can be constructed from plywood and framing materials to various heights and specifications. It is common to build a series of boxes of various heights from 6 inches to 36 inches in 8- to 12-inch increments, depending on athletic ability and the goals of the training program. It is optimal to have a variety of box heights to match athletic ability. You can build these boxes as a do-it-yourself project or purchase them from a training equipment supplier. Boxes constructed of wood can be heavy and difficult to move around, but they are also a very stable platform for jump training.

You can buy lighter metal-frame boxes of various heights for plyometric training. The advantage of metal-frame plyometric boxes is that they are easier to transport to training venues and are also easily stackable to minimize storage requirements when not in use. The downside of metal-frame boxes is that because they are often lightweight, they can be less stable for dynamic jumping activities. Additionally, boxes without side panels can allow an athlete to step or land through the open side on a missed jump and scrape the knees or shins on the top edge of the box. Lacerations and severe bruising of the shins and knees can be an undesirable result.

Newer plyometric boxes are constructed of a dense foam material covered in vinyl. These soft plyometric boxes offer the combined benefit of adequate stiffness and foam density for forceful jumps but softer edges that do not create injury if an athlete misses a jump. These boxes often come in various heights and can be stacked together via Velcro strips to create higher jumping platforms. Because these foam boxes are relatively lightweight, coaches and athletes should help stabilize the boxes when others are using them for dynamic jumps.

Plyometric boxes can be used for a variety of explosive and elastic lower-body exercises including static and countermovement box jumps, depth jumps, and numerous combination exercises with boxes and hurdles. The selection of appropriate box heights is critical for the safety of the execution of these exercises. It is always advisable to select box heights for jumps that are easily attainable, thereby minimizing the risk of injury.

Training Hurdles

For vertical deflection of an athlete's jump, hurdles can serve as a useful adjustable barrier. Regular track and field hurdles have traditionally been used for this purpose. While competition hurdles can be very heavy and expensive to use for plyometric training, particularly if athletes trip or fall on the hurdle during a session, training hurdles can be used. Training hurdles used by track and field athletes tend to be much lighter in construction and also tend to collapse much more easily should an athlete contact the hurdle during a jump, providing lower risk of a serious fall or injury. Hurdle heights should not be too high, allowing for the safe execution of multiple jumps over several sets. It is always best to select moderate-sized hurdles and simply jump higher over each hurdle rather than risk an accidental fall.

Hurdles specifically sold for plyometric jump training may be a more economical means of implementing a training program for multisport athletes. These hurdles are often constructed of molded plastic materials and designed for various heights, making it easy and safe to implement an enjoyable means of adding plyometric training to a group of athletes. If you're on a budget, constructing your own training hurdles with PVC pipe and joints can be a cost-effective way of creating a set of plyometric hurdles that are easy to transport and safe to use. A simple visit to the hardware store to purchase pipes, joints, a hacksaw, and some PVC cement can have you jumping in less than a day.

You can also use traffic cones for creating a vertical obstruction for plyometric training. Cones of various heights can be used with younger athletes, providing a physical barrier that they can jump over. Because a traffic cone is narrow, athletes may not always jump completely over the cone, allowing their legs to pass by the sides of the cone rather than over the cone. This is why actual hurdles may be preferred for jump training.

Medicine Balls

While much of the discussion on plyometrics has been on athletes launching their bodies over hurdles and up onto boxes, the throwing of an external object can be useful in the training of both upper- and lower-body plyometrics. Medicine balls come in various weights and sizes and can be used for explosive throws of all kinds. The balls themselves are often covered in leather or composed of a thick rubber skin that adds to the weight of the implement. Common weights for medicine balls are 4, 6, 8, 10, and 12 pounds. In general, lighter medicine balls are used for higher-speed throws, while heavier balls are used to develop power and dynamic maximal-strength qualities. Larger-diameter medicine balls with a greater surface area are often preferred for throwing and catching activities. Individual athletes can use bouncy rubber medicine balls for rebounding wall throws. However, some athletes prefer medicine balls with a dampened bounce quality, because a heavy ball with significant bounce can be hard to handle. Fortunately, there are numerous types of medicine balls of various sizes and compositions to fit to individual athlete and sporting needs in both indoor and outdoor environments.

Explosive throws with medicine balls can be carried out much the same as explosive jumps, with a choice of a pure concentric movement or the addition of a preparatory countermovement before the throw. Under both conditions, the weight of the medicine ball adds a load to both the eccentric and concentric muscle actions. For rotational throws, the gather phase, or countermovement, preloads the muscles of the core and shoulder before an explosive throw. Medicine-ball throws can also be combined with preparatory jumping movements to create a multijump pattern before a throw. In summary, medicine balls are a great tool for a comprehensive upper- and lower-body plyometric program.

Other External Loads

External loads can be combined with plyometric exercises to increase the forces during rapid movement. While a medicine ball is an implement that can be thrown or launched, other equipment can be used in combination with plyometric activities to increase overall load and enhance the effect of plyometric exercises. Take care not to overload by extending amortization and coupling times to a point at which detraining of the stretch reflex or overstretching of elastic components can occur. Ground contact times must be kept to a minimum, and preservation of the velocity of movement and technique is imperative under all loaded conditions.

Barbells and Dumbbells

One common means of increasing load during a plyometric exercise is to use barbells or dumbbells. Typically dumbbells are held in either hand along the sides of the body during in-place jumps. To use a barbell, hold it on the top of your back and perform jumps in place such as in a weighted squat jump. The key is to keep the barbell in contact with the back during repetitive jumps to avoid having it crash back down onto the vertebrae.

With both barbells and dumbbells, do not perform complex jumps or jumps onto boxes or over hurdles. Once again, the careful selection of loads for barbells and dumbbells is imperative for optimizing the contribution of such forms of resistance and maximizing safety. As with many technical velocity-based movements, more resistance is not always better. Finding the optimal load based on individual needs will yield the best effect.

Kettlebells

The use of kettlebells for dynamic strength training movements has increased in popularity recently. From the perspective of a plyometric program, repetitive kettlebell swings can produce stretch responses through numerous muscle groups in the upper and lower body as well as the core musculature. While it may seem intuitive to throw a kettlebell, it is not advisable because of the potential risk to other athletes and the damage that can be created by a heavy projectile in an indoor facility or a well-maintained grass or turf field.

Resistance Bands

Thick rubber resistance bands are commonly used for resistance of repetitive jumps either in place or over distance. For vertical jump training, resistance bands often are secured around the waist or upper torso via a harness, with the other ends secured to the floor. The bands provide resistance during the concentric motion of the jump but also can accelerate the body back to the ground faster than gravity. While this type of resistance can be a challenge, as with any external resistance method you must take care to ensure the resistance is not excessive.

With rubber bands, the resistance offered provides a performance result that is dissimilar to the natural force–velocity curve in jumping and throwing activities. Low- to moderate-resistance is always preferred in high-velocity movements. If too much resistance is provided during a movement that requires rapid acceleration or high velocity, the biomechanics of the movement can be significantly altered, resulting in a negative performance outcome.

For repetitive jumps over distance, use of resistance bands around the waist in partner drills can provide appropriate concentric resistance while limiting horizontal eccentric stresses that can overload the quadriceps muscles and lead to chronic knee pain. The same method can be used for medicine-ball throws, with a resistance band placed around the waist providing moderate loading during an explosive throw.

Weighted Vests and Belts

Weighted vests and belts have been used in jumping movements for decades, allowing for freedom of motion with a moderate additional load. Because you are not required to hold the weighted object, a weighted vest will allow you to carry out sport-specific activities with the added load. The addition of 10 pounds to a vest or belt, while seemingly not excessive, can prove to be a significant challenge over the duration of a plyometric workout. Weighted vests and belts are preferred over ankle or wrist weights because the load is situated closer to the center of mass. Ankle and wrist weights also place significant stress on the joints, particularly for dynamic movements.

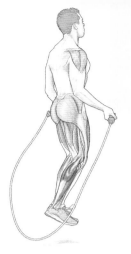

FOUNDATIONAL EXERCISES

When designing a plyometric training program, you have numerous exercises to draw on for your sport. In addition, every exercise can have multiple options for modification, whether for adapting to a specific sporting movement, combining multiple exercises in a series, or isolating a specific aspect of the movement to enhance its contribution to the overall effort. Foundational plyometric movements introduced to athletes in an initial phase of a training program help to simplify the process of teaching the exercises and also build the strength, power, and elastic qualities required for advanced training and, ultimately, elite competition.

Athletes often have a propensity to engage in training that is more complicated, choosing exercises that look innovative and intricate, as opposed to sticking with the basics. The danger in prematurely gravitating toward exercises that are complex is that basic technical skills can be neglected and necessary physiological adaptations diluted. Just as a foundation for a house must be strong, durable and balanced, foundational exercises must be administered in a manner that ensures that appropriate motor skills are developed, mastered and retained over the duration of an athlete's career. In the cases of plyometric exercises, this concept is made all the more critical due to the explosive and dynamic nature of the skills that are being introduced to athletes. Although the bulk of plyometric exercises tend to be oriented toward jumping movements, the physical qualities developed by plyometrics form the basis of dynamic, forceful movements such as sprinting, throwing and changing direction in numerous sports. If any key elements are missed in the physical training process and foundational exercises are not incorporated, the end product—regardless of the sport—will be compromised, with performance negatively impacted and the risk of injury elevated. Keeping things simple can often be the shortest path to excellence.

Following are key objectives for the establishing and implementing foundational exercises:

1. Provide building blocks for the development of more complex exercises. Before progressing to a series of jumps, you should begin with good technique in a single-jump effort. Single-effort foundational jumps or medicine-ball throws introduce less complex, acyclical exercises that you can master. Mastering basic qualities such as posture, foot placement, limb mechanics, and timing in less complex exercises can build both competence and confidence before you embark on more challenging movements. Athletes should not progress beyond fundamental exercises until all of these qualities are well established at a relatively high level of function.

2. Introduce achievable movements that may be deemed safer or less intense for less experienced athletes or in the early phases of a training program for advanced athletes. Jumps onto lower boxes or over lower hurdles provide an achievable goal and a safe environment for improving technical abilities and appropriate strength and power. Initially, these exercises can also be performed over reduced volumes in the form of a lower number of sets and repetitions to minimize fatigue and further improve technical proficiency.

3. Allow for the improvement of basic technique and mechanics through high-quality repetition of exercises over the duration of the training program. The repetition of foundational exercises not only improves the exercises themselves but also reinforces movement characteristics for other performance qualities being trained daily. Powerful hip extension on a box jump will reinforce this action for sprint starts, shot blocks in basketball, or tackles in football. The foundational movements should be considered a staple of explosive and elastic training that will keep you prepared and sharp throughout the year.

The concept of introducing and developing foundational exercises is critical to the success of a training program. While foundational exercises appear to be simple forms of more complex exercises, they are actually the building blocks of all athletic movement skills and human performances. A basic box jump may be viewed as a simple, explosive vertical jumping movement that spawns other exercises involving boxes and hurdles. However, the critical elements of a box jump from a static start or a countermovement jump have significant implications for how numerous other movements are developed in future training sessions. The posture, muscular involvement, and timing required for the execution of a maximal-height box jump are also involved in producing exceptional performances in a sprint start, hurdle jump, explosive medicine-ball drill, or countless athletic movements carried out in a typical sport training session. Refinement of these technical elements and physiological qualities in a foundational exercise can allow for a smoother and more direct transfer of basic movement skills to all aspects of sporting performance.

It is also important for foundational plyometric exercises to be viewed as a staple of all training programs—both beginner and advanced—that are kept within a training program for the duration of an athletic career and not discarded after a specific training or developmental phase. The key elements and qualities of foundational exercises can continue to be perfected and maintained for every athlete, regardless of age, experience, or ability.

BOX JUMP FROM A STATIC START

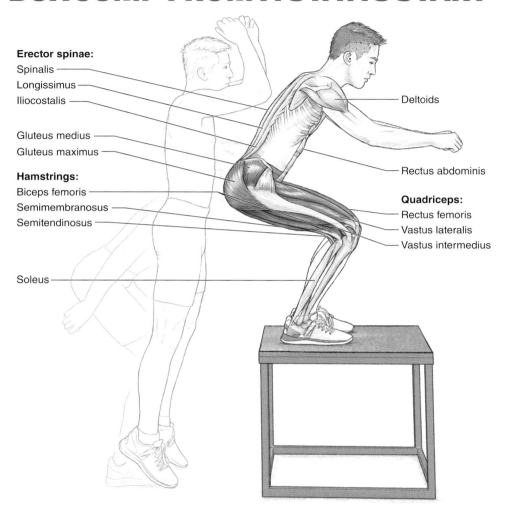

Erector spinae:
Spinalis
Longissimus
Iliocostalis

Deltoids

Gluteus medius
Gluteus maximus

Rectus abdominis

Hamstrings:
Biceps femoris
Semimembranosus
Semitendinosus

Quadriceps:
Rectus femoris
Vastus lateralis
Vastus intermedius

Soleus

Execution

1. Start with your feet approximately hip-width apart and knees bent in a partial squat position. Your feet may be slightly externally rotated depending on your individual needs and hip flexibility. Knees should be bent 100 to 140 degrees, depending on your sporting requirements. Torso is over the feet to ensure the body weight is shifted forward before initiation of the jump. Arms dangle beside the body, perpendicular to the floor. Stand with a neutral spine.

2. Initiate the movement by explosively producing downward vertical force into the ground through the legs and driving the arms forward and up. Ensure all movement is directed upward, with no countermovement or gather phase. As the motion progresses from a squat to a fully extended position, the back moves to an upright posture.

3. To prepare to land on top of the box, pull the knees up to an appropriate height to achieve a safe landing. Once the feet meet the top of the box, flex the knees and hips to absorb the force of the landing and soften the impact. Finish with your arms in front of your body to keep your weight shifted forward.

Muscles Involved

Primary: Gluteus maximus, gluteus medius, quadriceps (rectus femoris, vastus lateralis, vastus intermedius, vastus medialis), hamstrings (biceps femoris, semi-tendinosus, semimembranosus).

Secondary: Erector spinae (spinalis, longissimus, iliocostalis), deltoids, rectus abdominis, iliopsoas, soleus.

Exercise Notes

The box jump is a good exercise to use in the initial stages of a plyometric training program. Single jumps up onto a box of appropriate height teach proper starting posture, effective hip extension, and basic landing mechanics. Start with the knees bent enough to derive adequate power for the jump but not so deep it slows down the initial movement. Your torso should be over your feet to ensure a good portion of body weight is shifted forward, with the back in a strong, neutral position in preparation for an explosive movement. Keeping the arms beside the body provides enough range of motion through which to swing the arms for a powerful upward movement, extending the length of the body to the top of the box. Head position should be in line with the spine, with the eyes looking up above the top of the box. The flight path of the jump goes up and over the surface of the box, resulting in a soft landing absorbed by the muscles around the ankles, knees, and hips. Always choose a box height that is easily attainable over the duration of the training session. A box height that is difficult to achieve in earlier sets may become a hazard in the latter sets of an exercise.

VARIATIONS

Box Jump With Single-Leg Landing

When you master the bilateral box jump, you can increase the complexity of the exercise by landing on top of the box with a single leg. This modification adds eccentric loading to each leg but also challenges the balance and stability capabilities of each leg during a dynamic landing. Because the landing takes place on top of the box, it is less stressful than a single-leg landing from a regular jump or hop at ground level. The box height for a single-leg landing may be lower than that for a double-leg landing in the initial sessions with the exercise. As you acquire confidence and skill over time, the box height for single-leg landings can ultimately mirror that of a double-leg landing.

Weighted Box Jump

Attach a weighted vest or weight belt. Use a dynamic countermovement and powerfully swing the arms as you jump onto the plyometric box. Focus on the speed of the movement as you explosively extend the hips, knees, and ankles.

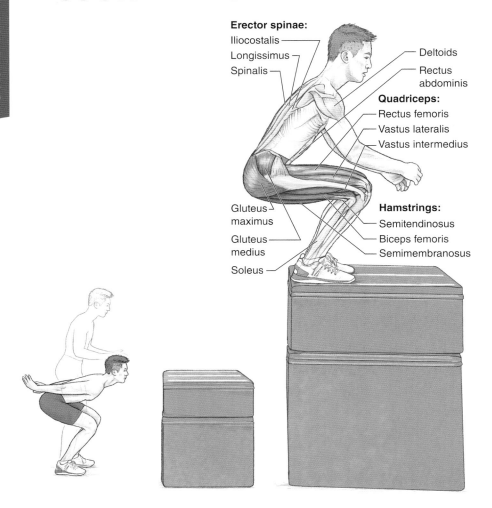

COUNTERMOVEMENT BOX JUMP

Erector spinae:
Iliocostalis
Longissimus
Spinalis

Deltoids

Rectus
abdominis

Quadriceps:
Rectus femoris
Vastus lateralis
Vastus intermedius

Gluteus
maximus

Gluteus
medius

Soleus

Hamstrings:
Semitendinosus
Biceps femoris
Semimembranosus

Execution

1. A box jump with countermovement begins from a much higher standing position than a regular box jump, with a fully erect standing posture for the starting position. The higher hip position at the start of the exercise allows for the downward acceleration of the body, calling into action the reflexive and elastic properties of the muscles and tendons of the lower body. The drop downward must be deliberate and fast, to the same partial squat depth used for a static box jump, with the torso moving forward over the feet. Arms swing back into a ready position behind the torso in preparation for the upward portion of the jump.

2. Reversing the direction of movement from down to up involves the downward application of force through the legs and the simultaneous movement upward of both the arms and the torso. Powerful extension of the knees and hips contributes to the jump takeoff.

3. You will achieve the landing at the top of the box by lifting the knees to an appropriate height. You'll achieve a soft landing at the top of the box by flexing the knees and hips, with the arms finishing on the front side of the body to maintain forward lead and balance.

Muscles Involved

Primary: Gluteus maximus, gluteus medius, quadriceps (rectus femoris, vastus lateralis, vastus intermedius, vastus medialis), hamstrings (biceps femoris, semitendinosus, semimembranosus).

Secondary: Erector spinae (spinalis, longissimus, iliocostalis), deltoids, rectus abdominis, iliopsoas, soleus.

Exercise Notes

The countermovement box jump is one of the more basic applications of a plyometric movement; the downward preparatory movement creates a rapid stretch of the primary muscles involved in the creation of an explosive jump up. The downward movement should be low enough to create adequate stretch in the muscles but not so low that it slows the movement and loses the elastic potential of the connective tissues. Ensure the downward movement is rapid, maximizing the contractile and elastic properties of muscle and connective tissues for the resulting jumping motion. It is also important to coordinate the timing of the arm swing to maximize the contribution of upward limb forces during the jump. When arm swing is not applicable, hold on to a medicine ball or simply cross your arms in front of your body to negate the involvement of the arm swing during the jump. This places greater load on the lower body and back for jump propulsion. The goal of the countermovement box jump is a maximal-height effort, easily reaching the top of the box. Maximal velocity of movement and speed to the top of the box should also be a consideration for each repetition.

VARIATION

Countermovement Box Jump With Rotational Landing

If you would like to add an advanced landing strategy for the countermovement box jump, use a 90-degree rotation on the landing at the top of the box. Because many athletic movements involve a rotational component, this variation on the countermovement box jump can prepare you for powerful jumping movements with a dynamic landing. Focus on rotating in one direction for each set of jumps or alternate rotation directions within a set. The objective is to initiate a powerful jump and land with a rotational movement in a stable manner.

DROP JUMP

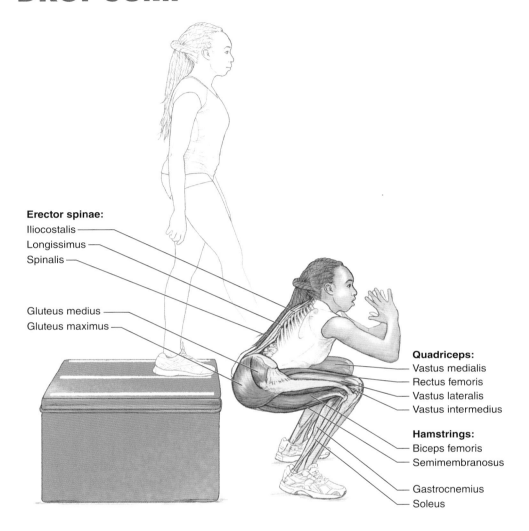

Erector spinae:
Iliocostalis
Longissimus
Spinalis

Gluteus medius
Gluteus maximus

Quadriceps:
Vastus medialis
Rectus femoris
Vastus lateralis
Vastus intermedius

Hamstrings:
Biceps femoris
Semimembranosus

Gastrocnemius
Soleus

Execution

1. Stand at the top of a low- to moderate-height box. Initiate the movement by stepping off the box, allowing both feet to descend to the floor evenly. Do not jump off the box because a jump can result in a much longer drop that may result in too forceful a landing.

2. While descending from the box to the floor, prepare for ground contact by slightly flexing the knees, hips, and ankles. You do not want to land these jumps with any rigid joints.

3. The balls of the feet land first, absorbing the initial forces as weight transfers to the heels. Once heel contact is made, the quadriceps, glutes, and hamstrings will handle the landing forces in a collective and progressive manner. The torso will come forward as the erector spinae muscles also decelerate the weight of the upper body during the landing.

Muscles Involved

Primary: Gluteus maximus, gluteus medius, quadriceps (rectus femoris, vastus lateralis, vastus intermedius, vastus medialis), hamstrings (biceps femoris, semitendinosus, semimembranosus).

Secondary: Erector spinae (spinalis, longissimus, iliocostalis), soleus, gastrocnemius.

Exercise Notes

Drop jumps are an effective means of eccentrically loading the muscles of the lower body. When weightlifting is not a practical means of developing leg strength, whether because of a lack of equipment or inexperience, drop jumps are a practical way to improve lower-body strength. Depending on the box height, landing forces can be several times greater than body weight. When initially performing drop jumps, use a low box and make a concerted effort to learn proper bilateral landing mechanics. Emphasize sequentially absorbing force through several joints. As you gain strength and technical proficiency through low drop jumps, gradually progress to incrementally higher boxes to increase training load. Heights of boxes can vary from 12 to 30 inches (30 to 75 cm) depending on ability and experience.

VARIATION

Drop Jump With Rotational Landing

Similar to a jump up onto a box, a drop jump can incorporate a rotational movement on landing to train you to handle both vertical and rotational forces on ground contact. As you step off the box, you can initiate a rotational movement with the upper torso. During the descent from the top of the box, ground preparation can take place for a 90-degree rotation. The landing will involve the same vertical deceleration process of a regular drop jump. However, rotational forces will add a new dimension to the landing, requiring greater involvement from stabilizing muscles throughout the lower body and core.

SQUAT JUMP

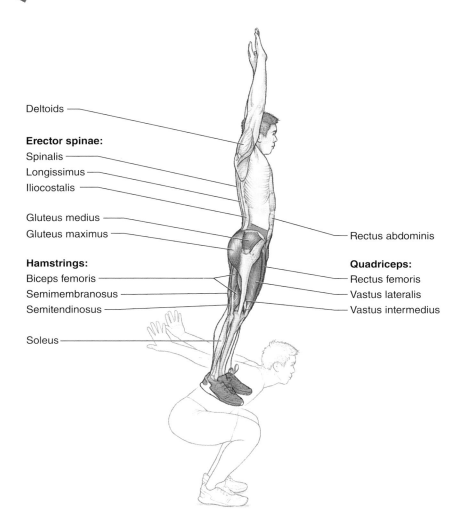

Deltoids

Erector spinae:
Spinalis
Longissimus
Iliocostalis

Gluteus medius
Gluteus maximus

Hamstrings:
Biceps femoris
Semimembranosus
Semitendinosus

Soleus

Rectus abdominis

Quadriceps:
Rectus femoris
Vastus lateralis
Vastus intermedius

Execution

1. Stand with feet hip-width apart and very slightly externally rotated to create a stable base of support. Initiate a countermovement downward to stretch and load the muscles and connective tissues of the lower body. The upper torso comes forward slightly to prepare for the takeoff. Arms can drop behind the body to prepare for the upward swing of the jump.

2. Simultaneously use a strong upward arm swing and hip extension to jump up. Back is erect. Your goal is to jump for maximal height. Prepare for the landing by slightly flexing the ankles, knees, and hips as you descend.

3. When landing, the balls of the feet will be the first point of contact, with the heels contacting soon after and a large proportion of the landing forces distributed throughout the thighs, buttocks, and low back. Once the forces are absorbed and the descent stops, return to standing and prepare for another repetition.

Muscles Involved

Primary: Gluteus maximus, gluteus medius, quadriceps (rectus femoris, vastus lateralis, vastus intermedius, vastus medialis), hamstrings (biceps femoris, semitendinosus, semimembranosus).

Secondary: Erector spinae (spinalis, longissimus, iliocostalis), deltoids, rectus abdominis, iliopsoas, soleus.

Exercise Notes

The squat jump is a basic exercise that involves no equipment and can be performed in place. As with the box jump, although the objective is to jump for maximal height, the landing forces are much greater in a squat jump because you descend back to ground level. In many ways, the squat jump combines the concentric actions of a countermovement box jump with the landing requirements of a drop jump. In each repetition ensure that takeoff and landing skills produce maximal concentric force and eccentric control, respectively. Even force application from both feet during takeoff must be accompanied by even impact absorption on landing. The squat jump forms the foundation for more complex in-place plyometric jumps. You can do squat jumps as individual repetitions or incorporate a pause between jumps to work on deceleration qualities and explosive strength for sport-specific skills such as change-of-direction movements. As strength improves, implement reactive or rebound squat jumps over multiple repetitions. These reactive strength and power abilities can also be developed using reverse overhead medicine-ball throws in cases where repetitive landings can be too stressful for developing athletes.

VARIATION

Lateral Squat Jump

A more sport-related version of the squat jump adds a lateral aspect to the jump. Instead of executing a strictly vertical squat jump, jump to one side and back to add lateral forces to the exercise. If a gym floor or field is available, perform lateral squat jumps over a painted line on the floor or field to provide a reference point. In cases where field or floor lines are not available, use a jump rope, dowel, or agility ladder to define lateral jumping parameters. The objective is to combine a maximal vertical jump effort with a lateral deviation to the side, landing with control and stability.

POGO JUMP

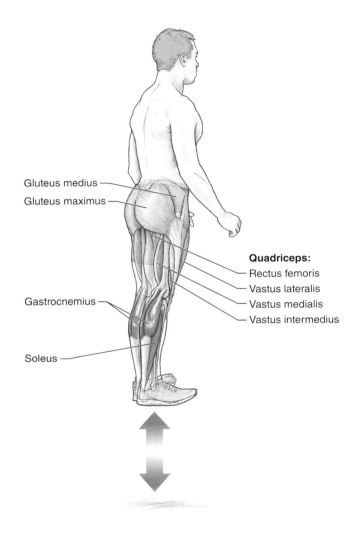

Gluteus medius

Gluteus maximus

Quadriceps:
Rectus femoris
Vastus lateralis
Vastus medialis
Vastus intermedius

Gastrocnemius

Soleus

Execution

1. Stand tall with the feet hip-width apart and arms along the sides of the body. Initiate the first jump with a short but quick countermovement effort. Drive the body up with maximal effort and maintain tall posture with the hips in line with the shoulders and legs for both the upward motion and the descent to the ground.

2. On ground contact, maintain a rigid body posture with only minor knee flexion to absorb the force of the landing. Ensure that the feet contact the ground evenly, with each foot dorsiflexed before ground contact to produce a strong, elastic response, producing a quick and powerful takeoff for the next jump.

3. Focus on high-quality, rhythmic jump repetitions of equal height, maintaining optimal body posture and rigidity over each set of jumps.

Muscles Involved

Primary: Soleus, gastrocnemius.

Secondary: Gluteus maximus, gluteus medius, quadriceps (rectus femoris, vastus lateralis, vastus intermedius, vastus medialis).

Exercise Notes

The pogo jump is a good foundational exercise for developing ground reaction forces and total-body integrity during elastic movements. The rebounding nature of the pogo jump lends itself to many sport movements, including running, sprinting, and changing direction. Maintaining an even rhythm over sets of jumps establishes a cyclical pattern of ground contacts—much like a pogo stick—that can transfer to other athletic movements. While the actions of the lower-leg muscles are critical for maximizing the elastic response for these jumps, the development of the rigidity of whole-body musculature also plays an important role in maintaining stiffness and minimizing the dissipation of kinetic energy through the body.

VARIATION

Lateral Pogo Jump

Pogo jumps with lateral deviations also help improve ground reactivity for agility movements in numerous sports. The side-to-side rebounding action of lateral pogo jumps also strengthens the ankles, minimizing the probability of ankle ligament sprains. You can perform jumps over a painted line on a field or court or over a very short hurdle to maintain consistency of jump height and lateral displacement.

ROPE JUMP

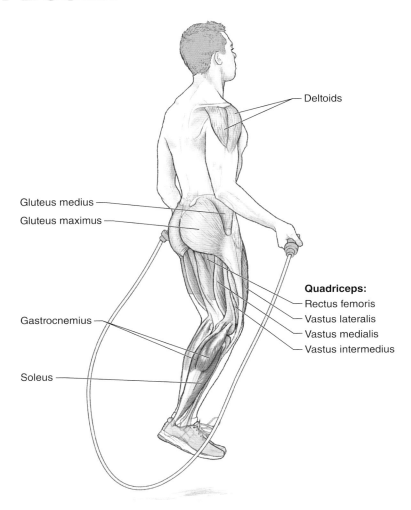

Deltoids

Gluteus medius

Gluteus maximus

Quadriceps:
Rectus femoris
Vastus lateralis
Vastus medialis
Vastus intermedius

Gastrocnemius

Soleus

Execution

1. After choosing an appropriately-sized jump rope, begin with the rope behind the heels and swing it over the head to the front side of the body.

2. As the rope descends to the ground, initiate a relatively small vertical jump over the swinging rope as it strikes the ground just in front of the feet. A rhythmic double jump can occur between each revolution of the rope, with relatively short ground contacts for each jump.

3. The frequency of rope revolutions and double jumps can vary based on your desire or training goals. A faster rate of jumps and rope revolutions can correspond with shorter and quicker ground contacts, while a slower pace may be associated with higher jumps.

Muscles Involved

Primary: Soleus, gastrocnemius.

Secondary: Gluteus maximus, gluteus medius, quadriceps (rectus femoris, vastus lateralis, vastus intermedius, vastus medialis), deltoids.

Exercise Notes

Jumping rope is probably one of the more traditional forms of plyometric exercise that has endured the test of time. The practice of jumping over a swinging rope provides a relatively consistent jump height and rhythm that evoke a stretch response in the lower legs and feet. A typical means of jumping rope is through a rhythmic combination of double jumps between rope revolutions, although several variations can be performed depending on the objectives of the exercise. While plyometric activities are generally carried out over short durations, jump rope training has been traditionally used as an endurance training method. Shorter-duration, more explosive versions of jump rope can be used to develop higher ground force reactions in the lower limbs. However, jumping rope over longer durations at lower intensities can be a simple warm-up activity before more intense plyometric exercises.

VARIATION

Explosive Double-Revolution Rope Jump

A more explosive version of the rope jump exercise is two revolutions of the rope with each jump. This exercise typically requires a higher, more explosive jump with a greater rope speed to allow for two full revolutions of the rope. Several jumps can be performed in succession, with approximately 6 to 10 jumps performed in each set. The objective is to maintain a significant jump height for all repetitions.

JUMPING JACK

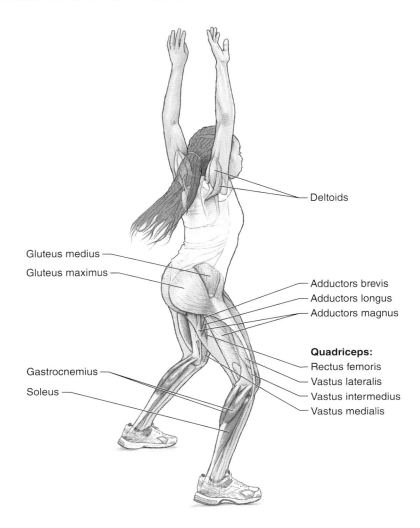

Deltoids

Gluteus medius

Gluteus maximus

Adductors brevis

Adductors longus

Adductors magnus

Quadriceps:

Rectus femoris

Vastus lateralis

Gastrocnemius

Vastus intermedius

Soleus

Vastus medialis

Execution

1. Start in a standing position with feet together and hands at your sides. Initiate the movement by jumping up and raising both arms laterally to a position over the head.

2. Land with both feet out to the sides of the body. With a reactive response on the ground, launch the body back up into the air, returning the arms and legs to the starting positions.

3. Continue the movement in a cyclical pattern, performing elastic jumps from a narrow stance to a wide stance, with the arms moving laterally up and down.

Muscles Involved

Primary: Soleus, gastrocnemius.

Secondary: Gluteus maximus, gluteus medius, quadriceps (rectus femoris, vastus lateralis, vastus intermedius, vastus medialis), deltoids, adductors (brevis, longus, magnus).

Exercise Notes

Jumping jacks are a classic repetitive elastic jumping exercise that can provide good general conditioning to beginner athletes who require an introduction to jumping exercises at a low to moderate intensity. Jumping jacks can be implemented as longer-duration fitness drills (15 to 30 repetitions) or shorter-duration (6 to 10 repetitions) elastic jumping drills. Because the jumps are of relatively low amplitude, this exercise is good for younger athletes and as part of a general warm-up for more advanced athletes.

VARIATION

Star Jump

A star jump is a more explosive version of the jumping jack. Instead of landing with the feet out to the sides of the body, the feet swing out during the flight phase of the jump and then back into the midline of the body for the landing. The arms also swing laterally up to form the midflight star pattern and then back to the sides on the landing. The landing of the star jump is also a rebounding elastic jump that vaults the body back into the air for successive jumps.

STANDING BROAD JUMP

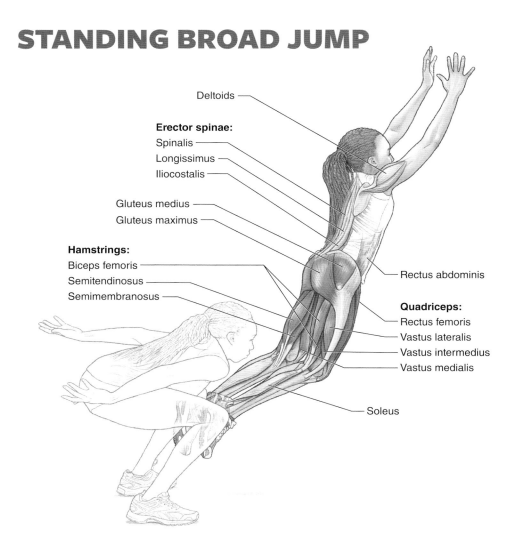

Deltoids

Erector spinae:
Spinalis
Longissimus
Iliocostalis

Gluteus medius
Gluteus maximus

Hamstrings:
Biceps femoris
Semitendinosus
Semimembranosus

Rectus abdominis

Quadriceps:
Rectus femoris
Vastus lateralis
Vastus intermedius
Vastus medialis

Soleus

Execution

1. Stand with the feet hip-width apart and facing forward. Arms can be held in front of the body in preparation for a backswing gather before the jump. Descend to a partial squat position with the torso leaning forward and the arms gathering behind the body.

2. Initiate the jump with a combination of a forward and upward trajectory of 40 to 45 degrees. Drive the arms in front of the body to a height above the shoulders, extending the hips into the initial flight phase of the jump.

3. In preparation for landing, pull the knees up and forward in front of the body, with the feet leading as the ground approaches. On landing, absorb the forces through the feet, ankles, knees, hips, and back in a progressive manner. Arms finish in front of the body to keep the center of mass forward, preventing a backward fall.

Muscles Involved

Primary: Gluteus maximus, gluteus medius, quadriceps (rectus femoris, vastus lateralis, vastus intermedius, vastus medialis), hamstrings (biceps femoris, semitendinosus, semimembranosus).

Secondary: Erector spinae (spinalis, longissimus, iliocostalis), deltoids, rectus abdominis, iliopsoas, soleus.

Exercise Notes

A standing broad jump incorporates maximal effort to achieve both height and horizontal distance. Although the broad jump is evaluated through a measure of jump distance, achieving adequate vertical height on the jump is also important for a good performance. Establishing an optimal jump trajectory takes some technical practice and is influenced by body posture and arm swing. When combined with a powerful leg drive, a vigorous arm swing can establish significant vertical force to elevate the body. Because the standing broad jump combines both vertical and horizontal forces, the forces acting on the body during the landing phase can be significant. Greater stress is placed on the quadriceps on landing due to the need to decelerate the horizontal momentum of the body. Take special care when programming and planning for broad jumps because of the additional stresses placed on both the lower body and back on landings. Standing broad jumps may require lower total volumes of jumps and greater recovery between sets than jumps that are more vertical.

VARIATION

Standing Broad Jump With Elastic Band Resistance

To reinforce hip extension during standing broad jumps, attach a strong elastic band around the hips. With the assistance of a partner, place the band on the pelvis to provide resistance close to your center of mass. During the jump, the resistance provided by the partner should be strong enough to force you to exert maximal effort on the takeoff but not so strong that it limits hip extension. The use of an elastic band also helps to reduce horizontal landing stress, allowing for a higher volume of jumps in a session.

ALTERNATE-LEG BOUNDING

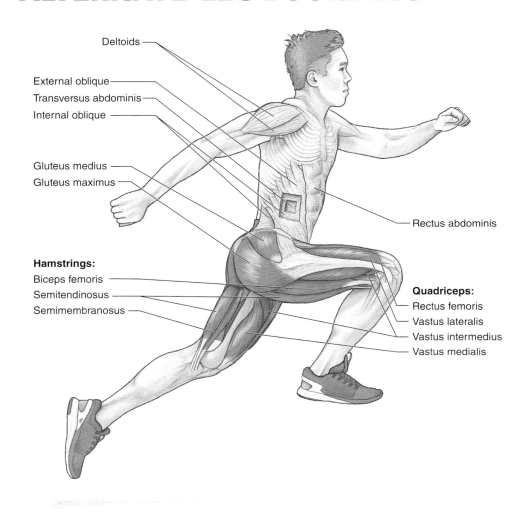

Deltoids

External oblique
Transversus abdominis
Internal oblique

Gluteus medius
Gluteus maximus

Rectus abdominis

Hamstrings:
Biceps femoris
Semitendinosus
Semimembranosus

Quadriceps:
Rectus femoris
Vastus lateralis
Vastus intermedius
Vastus medialis

Execution

1. Stand with feet together. Initiate the exercise by driving one knee forward, matching the effort with a single-arm drive with the opposite arm. The opposite leg will extend powerfully in an elongated stride.

2. During the flight phase, prepare the lead leg for ground contact and begin a powerful downward sweep with the intent of landing midfoot. Begin to drive the opposite leg forward to pass the landing leg on ground contact. Drive upward and forward. Swing the arms powerfully in opposition to counterbalance the action of the lower body.

3. Alternate elongated strides rhythmically over the length of the bounding set, driving for height and distance and maintaining short ground contact times on landing. The arm swing creates a rotational action between the shoulders and hips, generating force for powerful bounds.

Muscles Involved

Primary: Gluteus maximus, gluteus medius, quadriceps (rectus femoris, vastus lateralis, vastus intermedius, vastus medialis), hamstrings (biceps femoris, semitendinosus, semimembranosus).

Secondary: Transversus abdominis, internal oblique, external oblique, rectus abdominis, deltoids.

Exercise Notes

Alternate-leg bounding is a powerful version of elongated running strides. Bounding is used to build cyclical single-leg power for running, jumping, and multidirectional movements. A strong knee drive is critical for projecting the hips forward on each stride. Athletes are commonly told to attack the ground on each landing to generate adequate vertical and horizontal forces. To counterbalance the powerful rotational forces of the lower body, a strong single-arm drive is required. Initially, bounding on an uphill slope may allow for easier acquisition of technique. In some situations, such as for sprinters, bounding for horizontal speed may be emphasized, while in other circumstances, such as in the training of long and high jumpers, bounding for height is desirable.

VARIATION

Lateral Bounding

Perform bounding with a side-to-side motion to improve change-of-direction ability when multidirectional power is required. In lateral bounding, the arm swing travels across the body to counterbalance the lateral power delivered by the legs. For the initial sessions, a narrower lateral bound can condition the legs and ankles to prepare for wider bounds further into the training program. As with linear bounds, ground contacts should be short and elastic.

SKIPPING

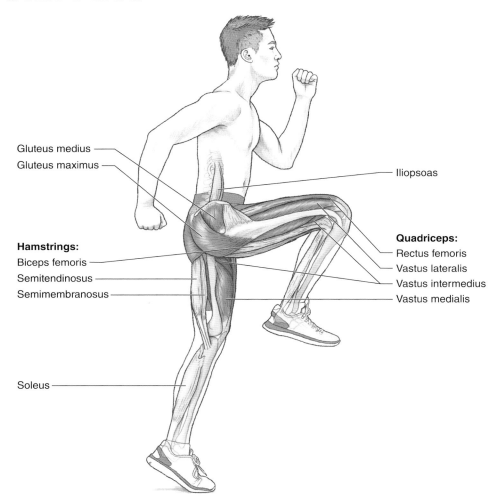

Gluteus medius

Gluteus maximus

Iliopsoas

Hamstrings:

Biceps femoris

Semitendinosus

Semimembranosus

Quadriceps:

Rectus femoris

Vastus lateralis

Vastus intermedius

Vastus medialis

Soleus

Execution

1. From a tall standing position on the balls of the feet, initiate the motion by lifting a knee and the opposite arm to the front side of the body. The knee should rise no higher than hip height, with the opposite hand rising to eye level.

2. The foot should descend rapidly to the ground to a position slightly in front of the body. As the foot strikes the ground, the opposite knee rises rapidly to a point even with the height of the hip. The arms drive up and down in opposition to the legs to counter rotational forces produced by the lower body.

3. Perform the skip rhythmically, with the feet providing elastic ground contacts on each landing. Each foot has a double contact with the ground before the knee lifts to prepare for the next skip.

Muscles Involved

Primary: Gluteus maximus, gluteus medius, quadriceps (rectus femoris, vastus lateralis, vastus intermedius, vastus medialis).

Secondary: Hamstrings (biceps femoris, semitendinosus, semimembranosus), soleus, iliopsoas.

Exercise Notes

Skipping exercises not only strengthen basic limb movements and improve whole-body posture for running and jumping mechanics but also train reflexive and elastic properties in the lower legs and feet for quick ground contacts. The skipping motion should feel light and quick, with the feet hitting the ground at a high velocity to vault the body up, maintaining a high hip position. The focus for the legs is on vertical force production into the ground, resulting in dynamic takeoffs on each ground contact. Arm action in conventional skipping follows the same path as the running motion, although skipping can be carried out with alternative arm actions such as circling motions, extended arm swings, or double-arm thrusts. Skipping exercises are commonly used in warm-up routines because they provide a moderate-intensity activation of the stretch reflex, preparing athletes for more intense plyometric exercises and movements in the main training session or competition.

VARIATION

Power Skipping

Power skipping uses the same posture and limb mechanics of basic skipping but involves greater force production for more vertical height on each takeoff. Focus on a combination of a powerful knee drive and rapid hip extension to create significant height on each skip. On landing, the objective is to rapidly initiate another takeoff movement in a coordinated fashion with an emphasis on downward vertical force with the takeoff foot and a powerful upward motion with the free leg and arm.

STAIR JUMP

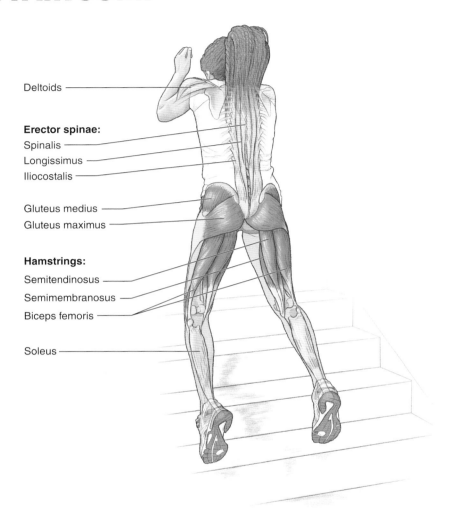

Deltoids

Erector spinae:
Spinalis
Longissimus
Iliocostalis

Gluteus medius
Gluteus maximus

Hamstrings:
Semitendinosus
Semimembranosus
Biceps femoris

Soleus

Execution

1. Choose a flight of stairs or stadium steps appropriate for your jumping ability. Select the number of steps for each jump as well as an achievable target for total number of jumps.

2. Initiate a double-leg jump with the feet hip-width apart. Ground contacts should be quick and powerful, launching the body up to the next target step. Arms drive powerfully up at each takeoff and recover in time for the next jump.

3. The series of jumps up the steps should be accelerating or at a constant velocity to maintain a consistently short-duration amortization phase on each ground contact.

Muscles Involved

Primary: Gluteus maximus, gluteus medius, quadriceps (rectus femoris, vastus lateralis, vastus intermedius, vastus medialis), hamstrings (biceps femoris, semitendinosus, semimembranosus).

Secondary: Erector spinae (spinalis, longissimus, iliocostalis), deltoids, rectus abdominis, iliopsoas, soleus.

Exercise Notes

Stair jumping is a common and cost-effective means of implementing consecutive explosive jumps with reduced landing impact forces. The jumps are essentially a series of takeoffs that maximally load you concentrically but moderately load you eccentrically. For this reason, stair jumping is an effective way to develop explosive power in the early phases of a training program. A set of 6 to 10 consecutive jumps can load you effectively without creating excessive fatigue provided that adequate time is taken between sets. As you get stronger, more steps can be traversed in a single jump, thereby increasing the concentric load. Do not try to jump outside of your capabilities because serious injury can occur if a step is missed. Once you establish a good base of concentric strength through stair jumping, the plyometric exercise program can transition to jumping over level ground, where eccentric forces will be greater.

VARIATION

Single-Leg Stair Hop

A simple way to increase load on the legs without jumping a greater number of steps is with single-leg stair hops. Single-leg stair hops can proceed over single steps to enhance lower-leg and foot strength, maximizing force production and minimizing ground contact time. Initially, to disperse load between both legs, perform hopping combinations for individual sets. For example, follow a pattern of two hops per leg, with two hops on the right leg and then two hops on the left leg, alternating back and forth for 10 jumps per leg. Single-leg stair hop combinations also build coordination and single-leg stability for change-of-direction movements.

47

LOW- TO MEDIUM-HURDLE JUMP

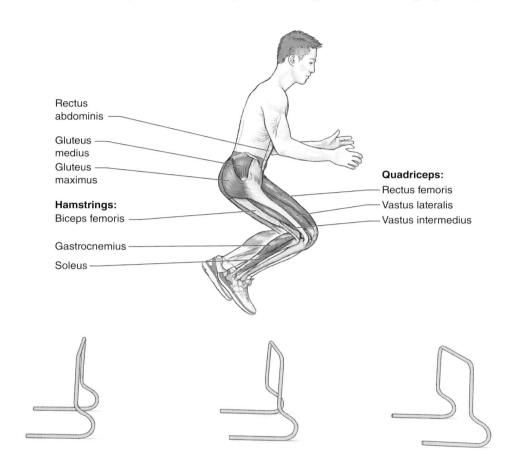

Rectus
abdominis

Gluteus
medius

Gluteus
maximus

Hamstrings:
Biceps femoris

Gastrocnemius

Soleus

Quadriceps:
Rectus femoris

Vastus lateralis

Vastus intermedius

Execution

1. Select a series of hurdles that are no higher than 12 inches. Arrange the hurdles approximately 2 to 3 feet apart, with 6 to 12 hurdles aligned in a row.

2. Perform two-foot jumps over the hurdles with minimal knee flexion on ground contact and during the flight phase over the hurdle. Arms can swing to the front of the body on each jump effort, gathering behind the body in anticipation of the next jump.

3. Ground contacts on landings should be light and quick, making use of the elastic properties of the lower legs and feet. Posture throughout the series of hurdle jumps should be tall and relatively rigid.

Muscles Involved

Primary: Gluteus maximus, gluteus medius, quadriceps (rectus femoris, vastus lateralis, vastus intermedius, vastus medialis), soleus, gastrocnemius.

Secondary: Rectus abdominis, iliopsoas, hamstrings (biceps femoris, semitendinosus, semimembranosus).

Exercise Notes

Low to medium hurdles provide a tangible barrier that deflects you vertically and ensures that you jump a consistent height and distance throughout the exercise. As in the pogo jump, lower-leg reactivity and whole-body rigidity are important for crisp and elastic ground contacts between each hurdle. Upper-body involvement, including the arm swing, can be minimal because the focus is on lower-leg stiffness and reactivity. Minimal knee flexion is required for both the landing and flight phases of the jumps. If you are bending your knees excessively in either of these phases, lower the hurdles appropriately.

VARIATION

Lateral Low-Hurdle Jump

Arrange low hurdles in a line to allow multiple lateral jumps back and forth over the hurdles. Jump laterally and rebound, progressing along the length of the hurdles.

MEDICINE-BALL CHEST PASS

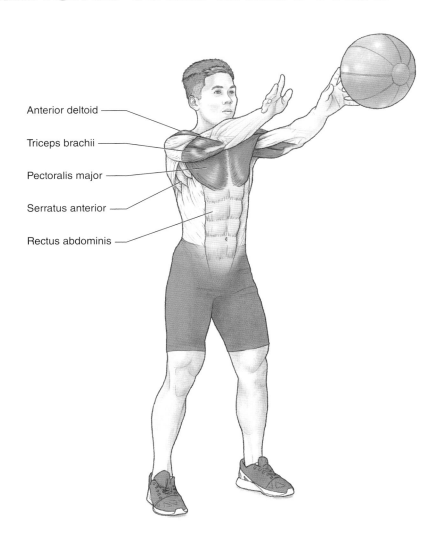

Anterior deltoid

Triceps brachii

Pectoralis major

Serratus anterior

Rectus abdominis

Execution

1. From a tall standing position with feet hip-width apart, draw the medicine ball in toward the lower portion of the chest and push the ball out powerfully to a partner or against a firm wall. Choose a distance between the wall and you or a partner and you that allows a strong throw that does not bounce on the ground.

2. When catching the medicine ball, absorb the incoming force of the medicine ball and then reverse the direction of the ball to a partner or the wall. In the case of a wall throw, the medicine ball rebounds off the wall and is immediately returned for the next throw. Partner throws should simulate this quick return and exchange of passes.

3. Maintain a firm posture throughout the exercise with a strong, stable stance.

Muscles Involved

Primary: Pectoralis major, triceps brachii, anterior deltoid.

Secondary: Serratus anterior, trapezius, rectus abdominis.

Exercise Notes

The medicine-ball chest pass is a fundamental upper-body plyometric exercise. The reactive nature of catching and returning a medicine ball builds both upper-body strength and elastic power in the chest, shoulders, and triceps and is applicable to many sports. Throughout a set of throws, maintain strong posture and core rigidity as well as a firm stance with the feet in contact with the ground. Any softness in posture will negatively affect the power and velocity of the throw. In the early stages of a program, use a higher number of throws (10 to 15 repetitions per set) to develop general strength. As the program progresses, use a lower number of throws (4 to 8 repetitions) to develop velocity and power.

VARIATION

Squat to Chest Pass

The addition of a squat between throws helps to build lower-body strength in coordination with upper-body strength and power. After catching the medicine ball, descend to the floor in a deep squat, keeping the medicine ball in front of the body. As you ascend to a tall standing position, throw the medicine ball to a partner or against a wall, using some of the momentum generated as you rise from the squat. With both partner throws and wall throws, be close together to ensure the returning ball arrives at chest height with good velocity.

MEDICINE-BALL OVERHEAD PASS

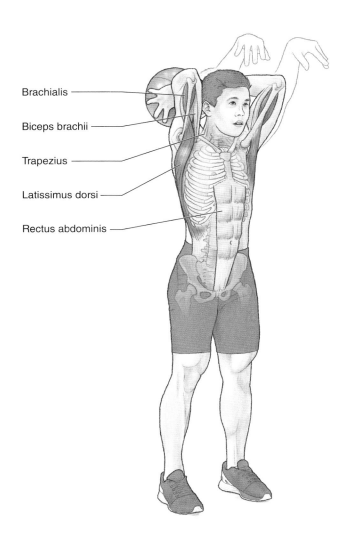

Brachialis

Biceps brachii

Trapezius

Latissimus dorsi

Rectus abdominis

Execution

1. Begin in a tall standing position with feet hip-width apart. Hold the medicine ball with both hands in front of the chest. Draw the medicine ball behind the head and then pass powerfully to a partner or against a firm wall. For the initial sessions, choose a lighter medicine ball and a closer distance between partners or a wall to allow for easier passes.

2. Catch the medicine ball above the head and allow the ball to draw the hands back behind the head to load the primary muscles to stretch in preparation for the next throw. For wall throws, stand close enough to the wall to receive the rebounding ball above the head.

3. Maintain a firm posture throughout the exercise with a strong, stable stance.

Muscles Involved

Primary: Latissimus dorsi, brachialis.

Secondary: Rectus abdominis, trapezius, biceps brachii.

Exercise Notes

A medicine-ball overhead pass is similar to a soccer throw-in. Select a ball weight that is not too heavy because forceful movements above and behind the head can be very stressful on the shoulders. When doing this exercise with a partner, get close to allow the passes to be caught overhead to maintain the continuity of the exercise. Similarly, when throwing the ball against a wall from the overhead position, being close to the wall will allow for a smooth flight path for the ball, receiving it above the head and enabling a continuous passing rhythm. Postural integrity and rigidity during the exercise are also important, making use of core musculature to stabilize the body.

VARIATION

Lunging Overhead Pass

You can also perform this exercise by finishing into a lunge position. The throw begins similarly to a regular overhead pass but finishes with the momentum of the throw carrying the athlete into a lunge position. After the release of the throw, push the body back into an upright position to receive the returning ball. The lunging leg alternates with each throw to work both left and right sides.

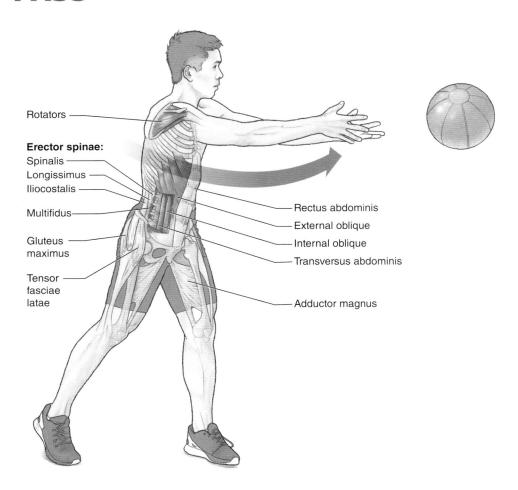

ROTATIONAL MEDICINE-BALL PASS

Rotators

Erector spinae:
Spinalis
Longissimus
Iliocostalis

Multifidus

Gluteus maximus

Tensor fasciae latae

Rectus abdominis

External oblique

Internal oblique

Transversus abdominis

Adductor magnus

Execution

1. Stand sideways to the direction of the throw with the feet shoulder-width apart and the knees slightly flexed, torso upright.

2. Draw the medicine ball to the far side of the body, rotating the shoulders relative to the hips to prestretch the muscles of the core.

3. Throw the medicine ball powerfully across the body with the path of the ball close to the abdomen. You can perform the throw with a partner or against a solid wall structure, choosing an appropriate distance to allow for powerful throws and safe reception of incoming passes. Follow through with the arms and shoulders on the release of the ball.

4. When receiving the ball from a partner or a rebound off a wall, catch the ball in advance of the body and rotate back to the far side of the body to prepare for the next throw.

Muscles Involved

Primary: Transversus abdominis, internal oblique, external oblique, multifidus, rotators.

Secondary: Rectus abdominis, erector spinae (iliocostalis, longissimus, spinalis), tensor fasciae latae, adductor magnus, gluteus maximus.

Exercise Notes

This exercise is valuable for the development of basic rotational power, particularly for throwing sports. A powerful lateral medicine-ball throw requires significant contribution from the lower body, generating force from the ground up. As lower-body power transfers through the core, the culmination of numerous muscular contractions results in a forceful rotational throw. Because rotational throws involve such a significant contribution from the lower body, this exercise also helps develop greater strength for multidirectional movement without creating overuse problems associated with excessive agility training.

VARIATION

Seated Rotational Medicine-Ball Pass

The seated version of the rotational medicine-ball pass removes the contribution of the legs to the throwing motion. Power is generated through the core musculature and the upper body. Seated rotational passes may not necessarily be used for developing power but can be helpful in isolating the muscles of the core and upper torso, particularly for higher repetitions.

EXPLOSIVE MEDICINE-BALL PUSH THROW

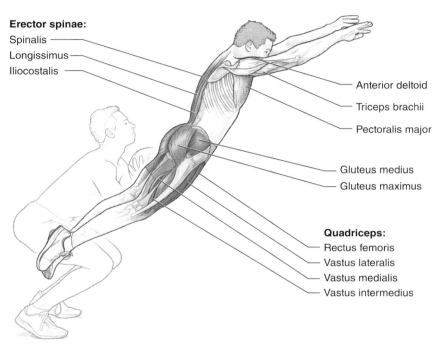

Erector spinae:
Spinalis
Longissimus
Iliocostalis

Anterior deltoid

Triceps brachii

Pectoralis major

Gluteus medius
Gluteus maximus

Quadriceps:
Rectus femoris
Vastus lateralis
Vastus medialis
Vastus intermedius

Execution

1. Hold the medicine ball close to the upper portion of the chest, with both hands behind the ball and feet shoulder-width apart. Descend into a deep squat.

2. Slowly roll forward onto the toes. As the body begins to fall forward, rapidly extend at the hips to launch the body forward.

3. Once you reach full extension at the hips, powerfully push forward with the arms to launch the ball at an angle of 35 to 40 degrees. Take a few steps after the throw to regain your balance and reset for the next throw.

Muscles Involved

Primary: Gluteus maximus, gluteus medius, quadriceps (rectus femoris, vastus lateralis, vastus intermedius, vastus medialis), erector spinae (spinalis, longissimus, iliocostalis).

Secondary: Pectoralis major, triceps brachii, anterior deltoid.

Exercise Notes

The explosive medicine-ball push throw is a good exercise for developing starting strength and power, particularly for sprint events in track and field and swimming. The rapid development of force from the ground through the arms also can contribute to contact sports such as American football, rugby, and ice hockey. It is also a good activity for warming up before explosive activities because of all of the muscle groups involved at such a high intensity. You can perform this exercise as an explosive throw back and forth with a partner or across a field or court with a small jog after each throw to catch up to the ball. Explosive medicine-ball push throws can travel 10 to 20 yards, depending on your ability. The goal is to throw the medicine ball with maximal force in order to achieve as much distance on the throw as possible.

VARIATION

Explosive Medicine-Ball Push Throw Into Sprint

Perform the explosive medicine-ball push throw as part of the start in a sprint effort. Once you launch the ball forward, transition smoothly into a sprint over 10 to 40 yards. Use a medicine ball of 6 to 10 pounds to overload the starting movement enough to provide a contrast to an unloaded start. Interspersing loaded starts with unloaded starts provides a benefit in the form of a more powerful starting motion.

REVERSE OVERHEAD MEDICINE-BALL THROW

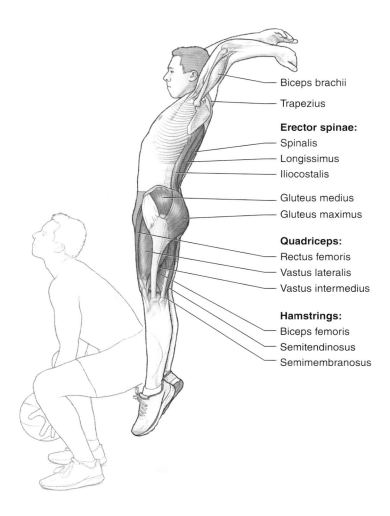

Biceps brachii

Trapezius

Erector spinae:
Spinalis
Longissimus
Iliocostalis

Gluteus medius
Gluteus maximus

Quadriceps:
Rectus femoris
Vastus lateralis
Vastus intermedius

Hamstrings:
Biceps femoris
Semitendinosus
Semimembranosus

Execution

1. Hold the medicine ball in front of your body with arms extended. Stand with feet shoulder-width apart. Descend into a squat, lowering the medicine ball between your ankles. The torso should be upright and the spine neutral throughout the squat phase.

2. Rapidly jump out of the squat, keeping the arms extended until you achieve full hip extension. If adequate force is produced from the lower body, the feet should leave the ground once the legs have achieved full extension. Once you achieve full extension at the hip, the arms can finish pulling the ball overhead.

3. Fully extend the body backward, driving the ball backward for maximum distance at an angle of 40 to 45 degrees. The body can displace backward with a few steps as part of the follow-through motion.

Muscles Involved

Primary: Gluteus maximus, gluteus medius, quadriceps (rectus femoris, vastus lateralis, vastus intermedius, vastus medialis), erector spinae (spinalis, longissimus, iliocostalis), hamstrings (biceps femoris, semitendinosus, semi-membranosus).

Secondary: Trapezius, biceps brachii.

Exercise Notes

The reverse overhead medicine-ball throw is one of the more commonly used explosive throws for training and evaluating power. The motion of throwing a medicine ball explosively overhead simulates the mechanics of a vertical jump. For athletes who require strength and power development before squat jumps or other more stressful plyometric jumps, explosive reverse overhead medicine-ball throws can prepare the muscles in a similar fashion with less eccentric impacts. This exercise also provides some tangible feedback on performance through measurement of throw distance.

VARIATION

Underhand Forward Medicine-Ball Throw

For this exercise, throw the medicine ball forward explosively with a scooping motion. Start in the same posture as the reverse overhead medicine-ball throw, but shift more weight forward during the explosive ascent. As the movement approaches full hip extension, the medicine ball will move farther away from the body until it is released in a forward throw. The full movement simulates a forward jumping motion, similar to a standing broad jump.

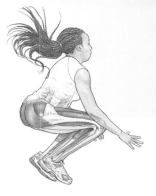

BILATERAL LOWER-BODY EXERCISES

4

A discussion of plyometric exercises almost always implies explosive and elastic movements that involve the lower body. A visual of an athlete jumping or sprinting is the most common representation of plyometrics, with the muscles and tendons of the legs propelling the athlete up onto boxes, over hurdles, or across a field. Because the lower body is the primary means of locomotion for the majority of sporting pursuits, identifying optimal plyometric exercises for the specific demands of a sport is imperative for preparing the lower body for explosive and dynamic performances.

In addition to locomotion, the muscles of the legs (figure 4.1) are required for landing, decelerating and changing direction. Training of these muscles must reflect the demands of various sports while not creating a situation where overuse of specific muscles and joints can lead to acute or chronic injury. Awareness of the specific muscles involved in a given sport and the relative involvement of these muscles in lower body plyometric exercises is critical for the development of an effective exercise plan.

While many of the same muscles will be used in all of the lower body plyometric exercises, it is important to understand that the subtle differences between one exercise versus another can be the difference in not only improving overall performance but also minimizing the probability of injury. The gluteal muscles, hamstrings, and quadriceps are all involved to varying degrees in lower-body plyometric exercises. The quadriceps are involved in extending the knee in jumping and sprinting movements, but can also play a key role in decelerating an athlete on a jump landing or direction change movements. The hamstrings play a significant role in powerfully extending the hip for explosive jumps and sprint acceleration but also flex and support the knee for many athletic movements. The gluteal muscles are powerful hip extensors for jumping and other explosive movements, and can play an important part in decelerating the body

4

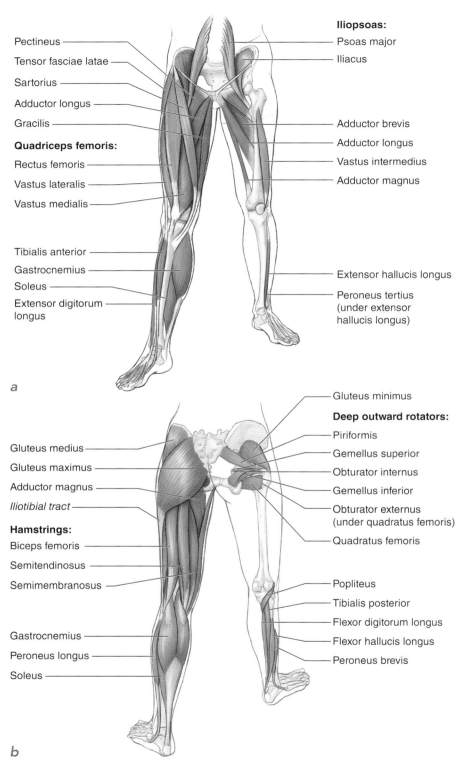

Pectineus

Tensor fasciae latae

Sartorius

Adductor longus

Gracilis

Quadriceps femoris:

Rectus femoris

Vastus lateralis

Vastus medialis

Tibialis anterior

Gastrocnemius

Soleus

Extensor digitorum longus

Iliopsoas:

Psoas major

Iliacus

Adductor brevis

Adductor longus

Vastus intermedius

Adductor magnus

Extensor hallucis longus

Peroneus tertius (under extensor hallucis longus)

a

Gluteus minimus

Deep outward rotators:

Piriformis

Gemellus superior

Obturator internus

Gemellus inferior

Obturator externus (under quadratus femoris)

Quadratus femoris

Gluteus medius

Gluteus maximus

Adductor magnus

Iliotibial tract

Hamstrings:

Biceps femoris

Semitendinosus

Semimembranosus

Gastrocnemius

Peroneus longus

Soleus

Popliteus

Tibialis posterior

Flexor digitorum longus

Flexor hallucis longus

Peroneus brevis

b

FIGURE 4.1   Muscles of the lower extremities: *(a)* anterior; *(b)* posterior.

during landings and agility movements. Below the knee joint, muscles of the calf can be involved in both high-speed elastic movements (gastrocnemius) and postural stability (soleus). The well-coordinated involvement of all of these muscles is what produces exceptional athletic performances for both training and competition.

Plyometric jumps involving two legs provide a stable means of loading the lower body with high-intensity explosive movements. It is common to initiate a plyometric jumping program with two-footed jumps for this reason. Bilateral jumps equally distribute and share the force of takeoffs and landings over two legs, making such exercises relatively less stressful than single-leg jumps. Once a foundation of bilateral jumps is built over a phase of training, single-leg jumps can be added to provide more complex movements and greater loads on individual legs.

It is not always the case that bilateral jumps are always less stressful than single-leg jumps. Factors such as jump height, horizontal velocity, and athlete coordination may influence the difficulty or impact of a particular type of jump. It is at the coach's discretion to determine the optimal exercises for a particular training session or a specific training phase for each athlete under his or her supervision. For beginners, it is advisable to take a conservative approach that incorporates basic bilateral jumping exercises for the initial stages of a program, focusing on the basic mechanics of jumping and landing. There are many different classifications of bilateral lower-body plyometric exercises allowing for a gradual progression of both intensity and complexity of work.

BOX JUMP VARIATIONS

Basic box jumps were introduced in chapter 3. More advanced box jump variations can be added to a training program as athletes gain skill, strength, and power. Box jump exercises are a valuable means to train lower-body concentric and countermovement abilities with reduced eccentric stress on landings. Adding resistance and complex movement to box jumps improves muscle recruitment as well as overall coordination and movement skill.

BILATERAL JUMPS IN PLACE

When specific training equipment is not available and space is limited, basic bilateral jumps in place are useful for developing both explosive power and reactive jumping. Unlike jumps onto boxes, jumps in place involve greater landing forces. The progression to jumps in place may require submaximal efforts initially to allow athletes to adapt to the landing forces over time. Jumps in place can also form a foundation of jumping exercises that eventually transition into jumps over distance, integrating a combination of vertical and horizontal force production.

COMBINATION JUMPS IN PLACE

Jumps in place can be combined to produce a pattern of movements that sequence through various ranges of motion and use different muscle groups. Combination jumps not only challenge strength, power, and metabolism but also force the development of a pool of movement skills that can transfer to a specific sport. In most cases, these jumps can be combined so you alternate, switching jumps from repetition to repetition. In other cases, two movements can be combined to create a more complex exercise. It is important to combine movements that are compatible and not beyond your ability. You should add combination jumps to a training program only after you have mastered the individual jump exercises over an appropriate time.

JUMPS OVER DISTANCE

Adding horizontal movement to bilateral jumps incorporates locomotion to lower-body plyometric exercises. If sprinting is considered one of the purest expressions of plyometric action, horizontal jumps can be considered a bridge between vertical jumps and fast running. Many of the same cues used in vertical versions of these jumps apply in horizontal movement scenarios. The combination of forceful ground contacts and appropriate foot placement ensures that horizontal acceleration can be achieved and horizontal velocity maintained with minimal braking forces, in some cases with significant height on each jump. Jumps over distance also give a sense of progress because they move through a set of jumps, whether it includes a measure of distance achieved or travel over a series of barriers. In the initial stages of performing jumps over distance, you can use submaximal efforts in a progression in order to develop the strength and skills for these exercises. Once a good foundation is developed, athletes can move on to maximal-effort jumps.

COMBINATION BILATERAL JUMPS OVER DISTANCE

Bilateral jumps can be combined to create an array of movements that challenge athletes both physically and technically. The intent is to arrange the jumps in a manner that forces athletes to adapt to exceptional takeoff and landing stresses, handling both vertical and horizontal forces. The combination of jumps arranged in training can simulate movement scenarios required in sporting events. For example, a basketball player may be required to jump forward quickly and then jump up to grab a rebound or block a shot. An American football player might have to jump over an offensive blocker and then explosively move laterally to make a tackle. These combinations of jumps can prepare you for the dynamic requirements of your sport by developing physical qualities and refining movement skills.

JUMPS OVER BARRIERS

While jumps in place and over distance can be effective in improving plyometric abilities, the use of vertical barriers encourages achieving and maintaining maximal efforts over consecutive jumps. As you jump over a barrier you derive a sense of achievement with each repetition. The combination of the incentive of jumping over a barrier and the sense of fun involved in traversing an obstacle course makes the use of vertical barriers an important part of a comprehensive plyometric program.

Historically, jumping over track and field hurdles is the most common plyometric activity over barriers. However, competition hurdles can be heavy and unforgiving if you occasionally miss a jump and collide with the barrier. Training hurdles tend to be much lighter in construction and can still be adjusted to various heights to fit the abilities of various athletes. When hurdles are not available, use traffic cones or foam cushions to create some degree of vertical deflection. The exact height of the barrier is not important, but the barrier should at least provide a degree of verticality to direct your flight path safely upward. In fact, it may be more effective to keep barriers at a height that does not encourage you to excessively lift your knees over the barrier. Learning to traverse a hurdle with limited hip flexion is more desirable because it maintains hip position over the feet and better prepares you for an efficient ground contact.

COMBINATION HURDLE JUMPS

Hurdles can be used in combination to create changes in both height and direction of jumps within a given exercise set. Low hurdles can be intermixed with higher hurdles to elicit variability in jump height. Hurdles can also have various orientations to direct you to jump forward or laterally jump. The variability provided in hurdle heights and orientations forces you to modify movements and adapt to the nature of the barriers.

DROP AND DEPTH JUMPS

Jumps down from boxes or raised platforms use gravity to impose loads on the body for maximal muscle recruitment on landing. In some cases, you can perform drop jumps to load yourself eccentrically, working on strength and landing mechanics. In other scenarios, you can use drop jumps from boxes to activate the stretch-shortening cycle and promote explosive reactive jumps up onto higher boxes or over vertical barriers. For all depth jumps, selection of the optimal box height is critical for maximizing positive adaptations for strength, power, and speed while minimizing injury risk. In most cases, it is best to err on the lesser side to maximize health. Many prescriptions have been identified for optimal box heights. However, because training responses vary considerably from athlete to athlete, biomechanics evaluation and athlete feedback are the best means of determining box height for these exercises. A gradual progression from submaximal efforts to maximal jumps, integrating an iterative approach, will yield the best results.

HURDLE AND BOX JUMP COMBINATIONS

Multiple hurdles and boxes can be combined to create a challenging obstacle course. The arrangement can incorporate jumps on and off boxes of various heights, along with hurdles of various heights interspersed between boxes. Arrange patterns of jumps that challenge the user without creating an unnecessary risk of injury. Predictable patterns and progressions of hurdles and boxes provide a good combination of moderate and high loads and encourage an even rhythm of movement throughout a set of jumps. In most cases, you should not exceed 12 repetitions in order to maintain the quality and speed of movement over multiple sets.

Variable Vertical Deflection Patterns

Arranged linearly, hurdles and boxes of various heights will challenge you to work between submaximal and maximal jumps efficiently. Developing a sense of control in the output of power and skill is an important quality for all sports. Specific arrangements can vary depending on your strength, power, and skill level. A box and hurdle arrangement may include a greater proportion of higher structures than lower structures if you're an advanced athlete. If you're a developing athlete, you may require a larger proportion of low structures, with only a few high hurdles and boxes periodically inserted into the arrangement.

Combined Vertical and Horizontal Deflection Patterns

A more complex arrangement of hurdles and boxes includes lateral jumps over barriers as well as lateral and rotational jumps on and off boxes. The exercise arrangement should not be overly complex. The idea is to create an organized challenge, not encourage risky movements beyond your ability. The integration of vertical and horizontal deflection can simulate both movement patterns and force requirements found in various sports. The objective is to elicit these responses safely and in an organized fashion.

Stair Jump Combinations

The use of a flight of stairs for multiple bilateral jumps is an easy way to incorporate multidirectional jumps of varying intensities. Because you jump up onto a higher step for the majority of repetitions, the eccentric load is much lower than with hurdle and box jumps. In this way, you can use stair jumps as a precursor to more intense jumps using boxes and hurdles. Stairs can be viewed as vertical obstacles that do not have the same eccentric stresses as hurdles or boxes.

You can perform stair jumps by jumping up individual steps or jumping up several steps at one time. You can also perform variable-intensity jumps by jumping one step first and then two or more steps on the next jump. Small markers or cones placed on the steps identify the target steps for these types of jump patterns. You can add lateral jumps along the width of the stairs or stadium benches, combining vertical power and lateral agility.

REACTION BOX JUMP

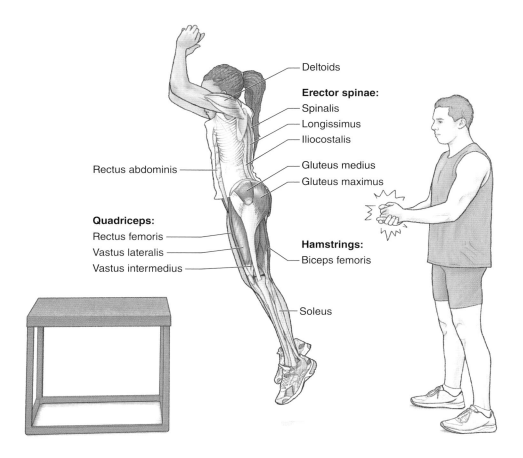

Deltoids

Erector spinae:
Spinalis
Longissimus
Iliocostalis

Gluteus medius
Gluteus maximus

Rectus abdominis

Quadriceps:
Rectus femoris
Vastus lateralis
Vastus intermedius

Hamstrings:
Biceps femoris

Soleus

Execution

1. Select a moderate-sized box that is an easily attainable jump height. Start in a quarter-squat position in front of the box, similar to the degree of knee flexion used in an athletic stance or ready position.

2. A coach or training partner provides a starting signal in the form of a hand clap, verbal command, or movement. At the signal, jump quickly to the top of the box.

3. The jump motion is similar to that of an unloaded box jump, with an emphasis on explosive extension of the hip, knee, and ankle joints. The emphasis on the speed of movement is critical for this exercise.

4. Jump to the top of the box as quickly as possible with both feet contacting the box surface simultaneously. Step off the box and assume the starting position for another reaction repetition.

Muscles Involved

Primary: Gluteus maximus, gluteus medius, quadriceps (rectus femoris, vastus lateralis, vastus intermedius, vastus medialis), hamstrings (biceps femoris, semitendinosus, semimembranosus).

Secondary: Erector spinae (spinalis, longissimus, iliocostalis), deltoids, rectus abdominis, iliopsoas, soleus.

Exercise Notes

Reaction box jumps can be performed with either audible or visual stimuli, allowing you to work on reducing reaction time and rate of force development for an explosive effort. For audible stimuli, a coach or training partner stands behind you and claps, blows a whistle, or shouts the command "Up!" or any other word of choice. Visual stimuli include hand motions, body motions, a ball drop, or a flashing light. In some instances, sport-specific audible cues or movements can be used for some sessions, while other sessions include nonspecific signals. Variation of stimuli will keep the sessions fresh and ensure focus.

VARIATION

Reaction Box Jump Off Touch Stimulus

To vary the reaction stimulus beyond visual or audible cues, use a touch stimulus. Before you jump on a box, a coach or training partner lightly taps your shoulder or low back to prompt the start of an explosive movement. A touch stimulus enhances body awareness and, when combined with an audible signal, conditions a profound response. A touch stimulus can be effective when introduced periodically with more conventional starting cues.

ROTATIONAL BOX JUMP

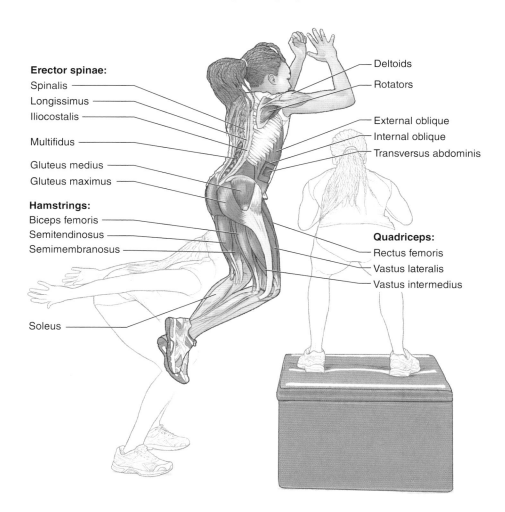

Erector spinae:
Spinalis
Longissimus
Iliocostalis

Multifidus

Gluteus medius
Gluteus maximus

Hamstrings:
Biceps femoris
Semitendinosus
Semimembranosus

Soleus

Deltoids
Rotators

External oblique
Internal oblique
Transversus abdominis

Quadriceps:
Rectus femoris
Vastus lateralis
Vastus intermedius

Execution

1. Select a box height that suits your jumping ability. This can be executed as a static start jump or a countermovement jump.

2. Initiate the jump with a strong upward motion delivered primarily by the lower body. An upward arm swing can accompany the lower-body push.

3. The arms, shoulders, and head, moving aggressively in the direction of the desired motion, initiate body rotation for the jump. As the upper body and torso rotate, the lower body follows.

4. The magnitude of rotation is determined by the orientation of the upper body. Rotation will be 90 to 360 degrees, depending on the specifics of

in the flight phase, the knees move up to a height at which the thighs are parallel to the ground at the apex of the jump.

4. As the body falls back to the ground, the legs lower to near full extension and the feet—dorsiflexed to provide pre-tension of the muscles of the lower legs and feet—prepare for an explosive ground contact. In anticipation of another repetition of a tuck jump, the arms gather behind the body. On ground contact, the movement is reversed into the upward direction.

Muscles Involved

Primary: Gluteus maximus, gluteus medius, quadriceps (rectus femoris, vastus lateralis, vastus intermedius, vastus medialis), soleus, gastrocnemius.

Secondary: Rectus abdominis, iliopsoas, hamstrings (biceps femoris, semi-tendinosus, semimembranosus).

Exercise Notes

The tuck jump is a dynamic exercise that involves successive elastic ground contacts combined with the lifting of the knees at the top of each jump. Although the jump is done in place, it simulates the muscular actions required for jumping over barriers such as hurdles. Hence, tuck jumps can be a preparatory exercise before engaging in successive jumps over vertical barriers. Emphasize short, powerful ground contacts to take advantage of the elasticity of the feet and lower legs. In addition, the efficient timing and coordination of the arm swing with lower-body jumping mechanics are critical in maximizing jump height. Because of the high-intensity nature of the muscular contractions involved in this exercise, take adequate recovery time between sets to maintain the quality of work in a training session.

VARIATION

Lateral and Rotational Tuck Jump

Once you have mastered the timing and mechanics of successive tuck jumps, you can introduce more complex variations. Lateral deviations on each effort simulate jumping side to side over a vertical barrier such as a bench or a line of hurdles. You can also perform tuck jumps with a rotational movement of 90, 180, and 360 degrees for each repetition. Starting a progression with 90-degree turns in each direction from jump to jump is a manageable means of introducing rotational tuck jumps. As you gain proficiency, you can incorporate greater degrees of rotation.

HEEL-RAISE JUMP

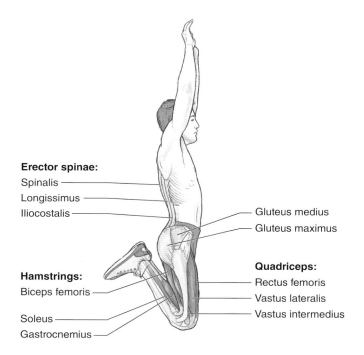

Erector spinae:
Spinalis
Longissimus
Iliocostalis

Gluteus medius
Gluteus maximus

Hamstrings:
Biceps femoris

Soleus
Gastrocnemius

Quadriceps:
Rectus femoris
Vastus lateralis
Vastus intermedius

Execution

1. Set up with the feet hip-width apart. Perform a strong countermovement downward to load the lower-body muscles and connective tissues then a strong upward arm motion to launch the body into the flight phase.

2. As you move up toward the top of the jump, lift the heels back and up with as much knee flexion as possible. At the top of the jump, you will achieve maximal knee flexion.

3. As you fall back to the ground, lower the legs to near full extension. The feet—dorsiflexed to provide pre-tension of the muscles of the lower legs and feet—prepare for an explosive ground contact. Initial sessions of heel-raise jumps can be performed as single jumps but can progress to shorter ground contacts for successive rebound jumps.

Muscles Involved

Primary: Quadriceps (rectus femoris, vastus lateralis, vastus intermedius, vastus medialis), soleus, gastrocnemius, hamstrings (biceps femoris, semitendinosus, semimembranosus).

Secondary: Gluteus maximus, gluteus medius, erector spinae (spinalis, longissimus, iliocostalis).

Exercise Notes

The heel-raise jump simulates the position that might be attained by a long jumper using the hang technique during the flight phase. The hips are pushed forward with the legs and feet trailing behind the body. A gymnast or freestyle skier may assume this position during an acrobatic jump or a specific skill. Exceptional mobility through the hip flexors and low back is required for attaining optimal range of motion and posture in this exercise. The jump can also incorporate quick, elastic ground contacts for repetitive jumps.

VARIATION

Lateral Heel-Raise Jump

A lateral heel-raise jump with quick ground contact can be performed in a similar fashion to jumping laterally back and forth over a short hurdle. The heel-raise technique keeps the hips forward and allows for a solid ground contact and transfer of force on each dynamic landing. This exercise forces the hip flexors into a lengthened position and reinforces tall posture during quick, elastic movements.

SPLIT JUMP

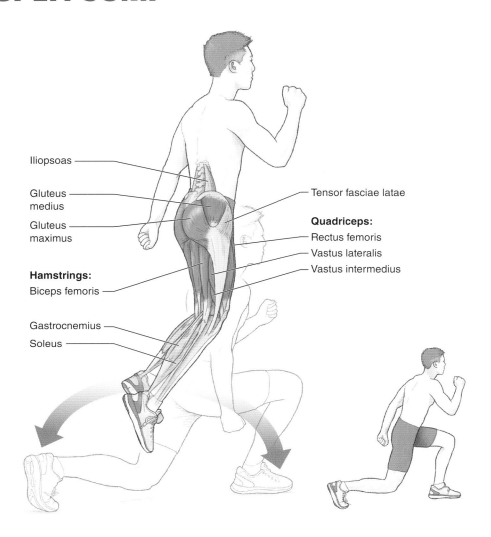

Iliopsoas

Gluteus medius

Gluteus maximus

Tensor fasciae latae

Quadriceps:

Rectus femoris

Vastus lateralis

Vastus intermedius

Hamstrings:

Biceps femoris

Gastrocnemius

Soleus

Execution

1. Begin in a partial lunge position with one foot forward in front of the hips and the other foot behind the hips. Do not separate the legs too much because this will reduce the amount of force that can be produced by the hips to generate an adequate jump height.

2. Perform a double- or single-arm swing with the arms moving in opposition to the legs to enhance stability. During the flight phase, the legs change positions to prepare for landing.

3. On landing, the feet assume the same range of split position established at the start of the exercise. The front foot lands relatively flat on the ground, and force absorption takes place through the hamstrings, quadriceps, and gluteal muscles. The rear leg lands toward the front of the ball of the foot.

4. Initiate the next jump quickly to take advantage of the elastic properties of the lower-body muscles, with the arms swinging strongly upward.

Muscles Involved

Primary: Gluteus maximus, gluteus medius, quadriceps (rectus femoris, vastus lateralis, vastus intermedius, vastus medialis), hamstrings (biceps femoris, semitendinosus, semimembranosus).

Secondary: Iliopsoas, sartorius, tensor fasciae latae, soleus, gastrocnemius.

Exercise Notes

Split jumps place additional forces on a single leg while the other leg provides some degree of stability and support. The front leg absorbs the majority of force in the gluteal and hamstring muscles with the rear leg supporting the weight through the quadriceps muscles and hip flexors (iliopsoas, sartorius, tensor fasciae latae). Split jumps also simulate a dynamic lunging motion used in numerous sports such as tennis when the player lunges to hit a ball. The exercise progression can include shorter ranges of motion on the split movement initially, transitioning to greater split distances as you gain strength and flexibility.

VARIATION

Split Jump With Medicine-Ball Rotation

Hold a medicine ball in front of the body. As you initiate the first split jump, rotate the medicine ball across the body over the thigh of the front leg. As the next jump is initiated, the arms take the ball in the opposite direction across the body and over the other thigh as it moves to the front. The ball continuously rotates back and forth rhythmically with each jump to counter the rotational forces created by leg exchanges.

SQUAT JUMP AND TUCK JUMP

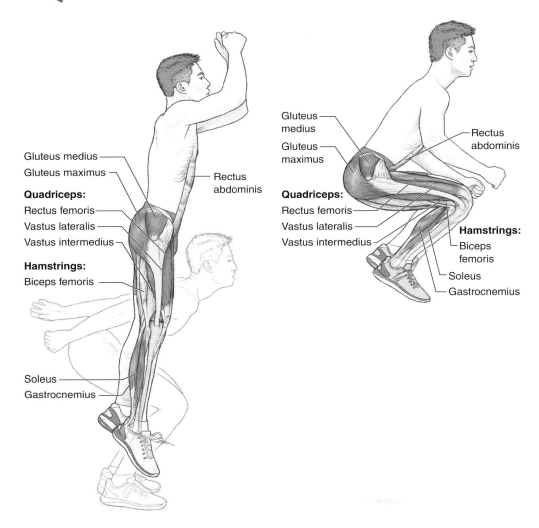

Gluteus medius
Gluteus maximus
Quadriceps:
Rectus femoris
Vastus lateralis
Vastus intermedius
Hamstrings:
Biceps femoris
Soleus
Gastrocnemius
Rectus abdominis

Gluteus medius
Gluteus maximus
Quadriceps:
Rectus femoris
Vastus lateralis
Vastus intermedius
Rectus abdominis
Hamstrings:
Biceps femoris
Soleus
Gastrocnemius

Execution

1. Begin with a powerful squat jump, driving for height and extending completely at the hips, knees, and ankles. On the descent, prepare for a quick ground contact, landing on the balls of the feet.

2. The landing quickly transitions to a powerful takeoff. As you extend upward, lift the knees until the thighs are parallel to the ground. On the descent, prepare for the next squat jump with a flatter foot contact than with the tuck jump.

3. The takeoff for the squat jump is preceded by a longer ground contact than the tuck jump. Drive up and extend fully through the lower body to achieve maximal height.

Muscles Involved

Primary: Gluteus maximus, gluteus medius, quadriceps (rectus femoris, vastus lateralis, vastus intermedius, vastus medialis), soleus, gastrocnemius.

Secondary: Rectus abdominis, iliopsoas, hamstrings (biceps femoris, semitendinosus, semimembranosus).

Exercise Notes

The alternating repetitions between squat jumps and tuck jumps require a different emphasis on both landing and flight mechanics. You will extend powerfully at the hip well into the flight phase of the squat jump, while the tuck jump will involve significant hip flexion at the top of the flight phase. On landing, preparation for the squat jump involves a longer amortization phase; the tuck jump preparations involve a more elastic, plyometric ground contact phase.

SQUAT JUMP AND STAR JUMP

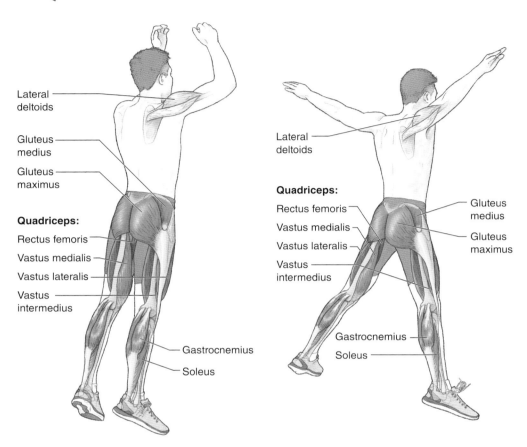

Lateral deltoids

Gluteus medius

Gluteus maximus

Quadriceps:

Rectus femoris

Vastus medialis

Vastus lateralis

Vastus intermedius

Gastrocnemius

Soleus

Lateral deltoids

Quadriceps:

Rectus femoris

Vastus medialis

Vastus lateralis

Vastus intermedius

Gluteus medius

Gluteus maximus

Gastrocnemius

Soleus

Execution

1. Initiate the sequence with a powerful squat jump, extending to a tall position through the flight phase of the jump. The landing of the squat jump
   will be similar to that required for repetitive squat jumps, with a similar
   ground contact phase and gather for the next repetition.

2. The next jump begins with the same takeoff emphasis, with the flight phase
   including abduction of both the legs and the arms to form a star shape at
   the apex of the jump. The arms and legs adduct during the descent phase
   in preparation for the next jump.

3. Follow the star jump with a squat jump, reintroducing a more conventional flight phase.

Muscles Involved

Primary: Gluteus maximus, gluteus medius, quadriceps (rectus femoris, vastus lateralis, vastus intermedius, vastus medialis), soleus, gastrocnemius.

Secondary: Lateral deltoids, gluteus minimus.

Exercise Notes

The combination of squat jumps and star jumps introduces a slight variation on the flight mechanics of the jumps, switching between a conventional flight phase and an approach that involves abduction of the legs and arms into a star shape. The abduction action recruits the lateral deltoids in the shoulder and the gluteus medius and gluteus minimus in the hips through the flight phase of the star jump.

IN-PLACE TUCK JUMP AND HEEL-RAISE JUMP

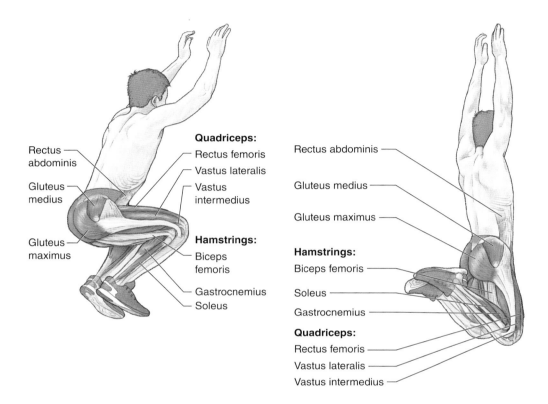

Rectus abdominis

Gluteus medius

Gluteus maximus

Quadriceps:
Rectus femoris
Vastus lateralis
Vastus intermedius

Hamstrings:
Biceps femoris
Gastrocnemius
Soleus

Rectus abdominis

Gluteus medius

Gluteus maximus

Hamstrings:
Biceps femoris
Soleus
Gastrocnemius

Quadriceps:
Rectus femoris
Vastus lateralis
Vastus intermedius

Execution

1. Begin with a powerful takeoff into a tuck jump. Lift the knees to hip level during the flight phase and then descend toward the ground in preparation for landing.

2. Land on the balls of the feet with a short, elastic ground contact to reverse the direction of movement back into the air. Move the heels back and up with significant knee flexion. The hips extend forward at the top of the jump.

3. Descend from the heel-raise jump by extending the legs back underneath the body to prepare to land on the balls of the feet. Use an elastic ground contact to vault back up into a tuck jump.

Muscles Involved

Primary: Gluteus maximus, gluteus medius, quadriceps (rectus femoris, vastus lateralis, vastus intermedius, vastus medialis), soleus, gastrocnemius.

Secondary: Rectus abdominis, iliopsoas, hamstrings (biceps femoris, semi-tendinosus, semimembranosus), sartorius.

Exercise Notes

The tuck jump and heel-raise jump combination provides a contrast between the flight phases of each jump: The tuck jump involves significant hip flexion and the heel-raise jump requires extensive hip extension. The rapid shortening and lengthening of the major hip flexors (iliopsoas, sartorius, and rectus femoris) during the flight phases simulate the demands placed on these muscles during many dynamic movements in sport. This combination jump is one of the more demanding exercises because of the maximal elastic nature of the jumps and the extreme range of motion experienced by the legs.

POGO JUMP AND TUCK JUMP

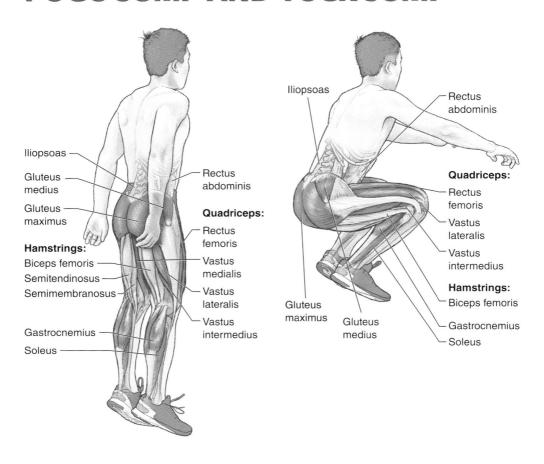

Iliopsoas

Gluteus
medius

Gluteus
maximus

Hamstrings:
Biceps femoris
Semitendinosus
Semimembranosus

Gastrocnemius

Soleus

Rectus
abdominis

Quadriceps:
Rectus
femoris
Vastus
medialis
Vastus
lateralis
Vastus
intermedius

Iliopsoas

Rectus
abdominis

Quadriceps:
Rectus
femoris
Vastus
lateralis
Vastus
intermedius

Hamstrings:
Biceps femoris

Gluteus
maximus

Gluteus
medius

Gastrocnemius

Soleus

Execution

1. Initiate the pogo jump with a countermovement of limited depth, emphasizing the contribution of the lower legs and feet. After each jump, land
   on the balls of the feet and use an elastic response to provide propulsion
   into the air.

2. After the pogo jump, perform an explosive tuck jump, lifting the knees to
   the height of the hips. The tuck jump involves more whole-body movement
   and greater intensity.

3. Descend from the tuck jump by lowering the legs to an extended position in preparation for the next active pogo jump. Maintain a consistent rhythm with quick ground contacts throughout each set of jumps.

Muscles Involved

Primary: Gluteus maximus, gluteus medius, quadriceps (rectus femoris, vastus lateralis, vastus intermedius, vastus medialis), soleus, gastrocnemius.

Secondary: Rectus abdominis, iliopsoas, hamstrings (biceps femoris, semi-tendinosus, semimembranosus).

Exercise Notes

The pogo jump and tuck jump combination is an effective way to introduce younger athletes to more complex jumping activities. Consecutive tuck jumps can be very demanding for younger athletes. Alternating pogo jumps with tuck jumps provides a break between more intense repetitions of tuck jumps while maintaining a continuous series of elastic ground contacts during a set. In many ways, this combination of jumps can simulate a low-hurdle jump preceding a high-hurdle jump.

CONSECUTIVE BROAD JUMP

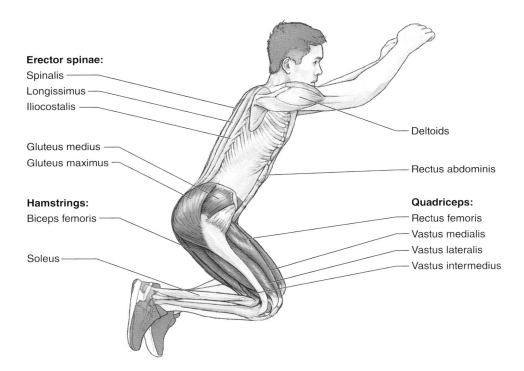

Erector spinae:
Spinalis
Longissimus
Iliocostalis

Gluteus medius
Gluteus maximus

Hamstrings:
Biceps femoris

Soleus

Deltoids

Rectus abdominis

Quadriceps:
Rectus femoris
Vastus medialis
Vastus lateralis
Vastus intermedius

Execution

1. Stand with feet hip-width apart and moderate knee flexion. Before initiating the first broad jump, use a moderate countermovement to create greater force production in the legs and a strong hip extension. Use a strong double-arm swing with the jump takeoff, driving the body forward and upward powerfully.

2. While it is important to emphasize horizontal distance in the broad jump, it is also critical to achieve a takeoff trajectory of no lower than 30 degrees on each jump.

3. Each double-leg landing occurs just slightly in front of your center of mass, conserving momentum and converting both vertical and horizontal force. The feet land relatively flat, with the landing forces absorbed in the quadriceps, gluteals, and lower back.

4. Consecutive landings and takeoffs involve moderate knee flexion, enough to safely absorb the landing forces and create propulsion for the next jump but not so much that you have losses in horizontal velocity and distance.

Muscles Involved

Primary: Gluteus maximus, gluteus medius, quadriceps (rectus femoris, vastus lateralis, vastus intermedius, vastus medialis), hamstrings (biceps femoris, semitendinosus, semimembranosus).

Secondary: Erector spinae (spinalis, longissimus, iliocostalis), deltoids, rectus abdominis, iliopsoas, soleus.

Exercise Notes

A set of consecutive broad jumps over distance is a strenuous exercise that involves both significant concentric and eccentric efforts. The intent is to achieve the greatest horizontal distances on each repetition without losing momentum over the entire set of jumps. The tendency to stretch the feet out in front of the body for maximum distance in a solitary broad jump is not as efficient a strategy in consecutive broad jumps because you would have significant braking forces. The goal is to minimize ground contact time and begin the next broad jump as quickly as possible. Greater horizontal velocity in these jumps typically results in greater overall jump distances. Because consecutive broad jumps can be extremely stressful on the legs and back, you should use relatively few repetitions (no more than six jumps in a set). In most cases, this would translate to a total distance of no more than 15 meters.

VARIATION

Broad Jump With Lateral Deviation

Although broad jumps are intended to achieve the greatest horizontal distance, you can incorporate a slight lateral deviation. You should still place a priority on linear distance achieved, with only a short distance covered laterally for each repetition. Performing broad jumps along a field sideline, crossing back and forth over the line on each repetition, is a good example of this variation.

SPLIT JUMPS OVER DISTANCE

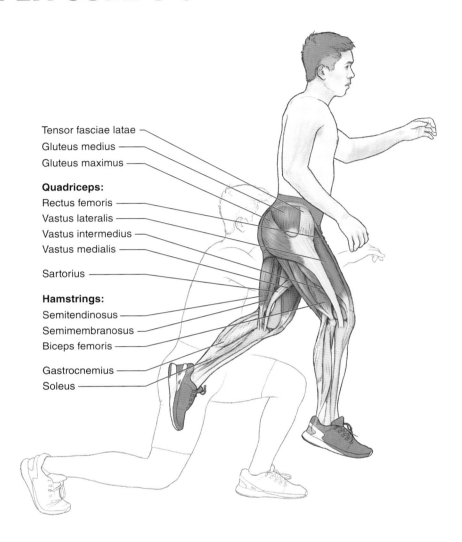

Tensor fasciae latae
Gluteus medius
Gluteus maximus

Quadriceps:
Rectus femoris
Vastus lateralis
Vastus intermedius
Vastus medialis

Sartorius

Hamstrings:
Semitendinosus
Semimembranosus
Biceps femoris

Gastrocnemius
Soleus

Execution

1. From a lunge position, initiate a split jump with an emphasis on both vertical and horizontal distance. During the flight phase, switch leg positions to prepare for landing, with the front foot landing relatively flat and the rear foot landing on the toes.

2. As in the stationary split jump, perform a double- or single-arm swing with the arms moving in opposition to the legs to enhance stability.

3. Keep ground contacts quick and light and the split distance between front and rear feet small.

4. Advance forward on each jump, emphasizing quick but stable ground contacts.

Muscles Involved

Primary: Gluteus maximus, gluteus medius, quadriceps (rectus femoris, vastus lateralis, vastus intermedius, vastus medialis), hamstrings (biceps femoris, semitendinosus, semimembranosus).

Secondary: Iliopsoas, sartorius, tensor fasciae latae, soleus, gastrocnemius.

Exercise Notes

Perform lunging split jumps over a prescribed distance, emphasizing both height and horizontal travel for each repetition. The progression forward can be quite slow with many repetitions achieved in a relatively short distance. Split jumps over distance can serve as a supplementary exercise for higher-velocity single-leg exercises such as bounding for power and speed.

VARIATION

Reverse Split Jump

You can perform progressive split jumps backward over distance to work on the same muscle groups in a different sequence. This variation challenges the muscles differently but also requires greater skill.

91

STANDING BROAD JUMP AND SQUAT JUMP SEQUENCE

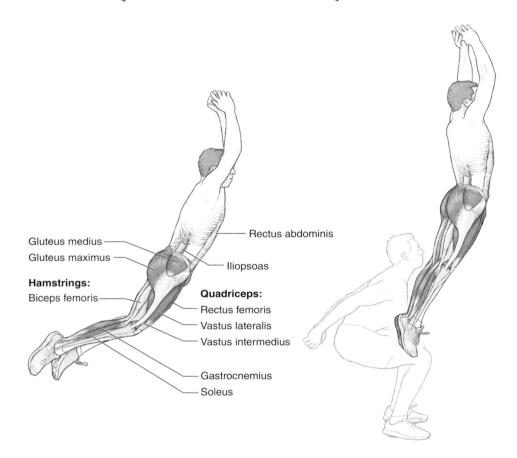

Gluteus medius

Gluteus maximus

Hamstrings:

Biceps femoris

Rectus abdominis

Iliopsoas

Quadriceps:

Rectus femoris

Vastus lateralis

Vastus intermedius

Gastrocnemius

Soleus

Execution

1. Initiate the sequence with a broad jump for maximum distance, combining powerful hip, knee, and ankle extension with a strong arm drive. Prepare to land flat-footed, absorbing the landing forces with the entire lower body.

2. Once the landing is complete, immediately drive the body powerfully upward, achieving maximal height in a squat jump. Land from this jump with the initial contact on the balls of the feet, settling onto the heels very quickly.

3. Explode forward into another broad jump, combining both horizontal and vertical force production. Complete the jumps alternatively in a smooth and efficient manner.

Muscles Involved

Primary: Gluteus maximus, gluteus medius, quadriceps (rectus femoris, vastus lateralis, vastus intermedius, vastus medialis), soleus, gastrocnemius.

Secondary: Rectus abdominis, iliopsoas, hamstrings (biceps femoris, semitendinosus, semimembranosus).

Exercise Notes

Combining broad jumps and squat jumps challenges you to achieve maximal horizontal distance on one repetition immediately followed by a maximal vertical effort on the next repetition. The conversion of horizontal speed and momentum into vertical force production and height is common in many sports such as basketball, volleyball, and track and field. Learning to perform these combinations of movements efficiently will transfer to many sporting scenarios.

FORWARD TUCK JUMP AND HEEL-RAISE JUMP

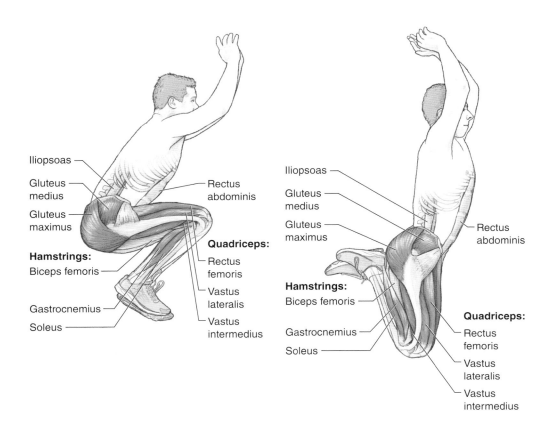

Iliopsoas

Gluteus medius

Gluteus maximus

Rectus abdominis

Hamstrings:
Biceps femoris

Quadriceps:

Rectus femoris

Vastus lateralis

Gastrocnemius

Soleus

Vastus intermedius

Iliopsoas

Gluteus medius

Gluteus maximus

Rectus abdominis

Hamstrings:
Biceps femoris

Quadriceps:

Gastrocnemius

Rectus femoris

Soleus

Vastus lateralis

Vastus intermedius

Execution

1. Initiate the jump sequence with a takeoff into a tuck jump moving forward horizontally. Bring the knees up to hip level during the flight phase and then descend toward the ground in preparation for landing.

2. Land on the balls of the feet and minimize ground contact time. Rapidly jump up again and raise the heels to the buttocks. Pushing the hips forward at the top of the jump, similar to a long jumper in a flight phase, facilitates greater horizontal travel on each jump.

3. On the descent of the heel-raise jump, prepare to initiate another tuck jump over distance. Each jump will incrementally advance over a prescribed distance. In most cases, this distance is 10 to 20 meters.

Muscles Involved

Primary: Gluteus maximus, gluteus medius, quadriceps (rectus femoris, vastus lateralis, vastus intermedius, vastus medialis), soleus, gastrocnemius.

Secondary: Rectus abdominis, iliopsoas, hamstrings (biceps femoris, semitendinosus, semimembranosus).

Exercise Notes

Performing consecutive tuck jumps and heel-raise jumps challenges you to combine different actions of the hip during the flight phases while also attaining horizontal distance on each effort. The skill required for efficiently completing these combinations of jumps is significant. Track and field athletes, volleyball players, and gymnasts benefit from the dynamic nature of these jump combinations.

STANDING BROAD JUMP AND LATERAL SQUAT JUMP SEQUENCE

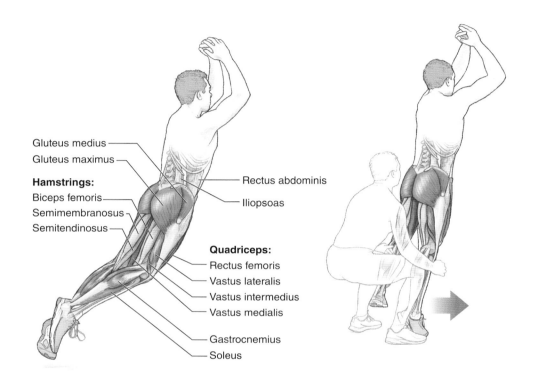

Gluteus medius

Gluteus maximus

Hamstrings:

Biceps femoris

Semimembranosus

Semitendinosus

Rectus abdominis

Iliopsoas

Quadriceps:

Rectus femoris

Vastus lateralis

Vastus intermedius

Vastus medialis

Gastrocnemius

Soleus

Execution

1. Follow a maximal broad jump forward with a lateral squat jump to the right. Knee flexion on the landing of each jump can be moderate to deep, depending on your strength level. A lower hip position will allow for a stronger and more stable change of direction.

2. After landing the lateral jump, initiate another linear broad jump forward, striving for maximal distance. Follow this broad jump with a powerful lateral jump to the left. Continue this alternating sequence for a maximum of 10 jumps total, although fewer jumps may be required.

3. With all jumps, keep the jumps under control, with very clean lines on each segment. If you begin to lose control, you may ingrain bad habits and compromise safety.

Muscles Involved

Primary: Gluteus maximus, gluteus medius, quadriceps (rectus femoris, vastus lateralis, vastus intermedius, vastus medialis), soleus, gastrocnemius.

Secondary: Rectus abdominis, iliopsoas, hamstrings (biceps femoris, semi-tendinosus, semimembranosus).

Exercise Notes

Maximal broad jumps combined with lateral squat jumps provide exceptional preparation for athletes who require multidirectional power and skill. The conversion of linear speed and power into efficient lateral movement is the key to success in many sports, including soccer, rugby, American football, and basketball. Multiple combinations of linear and lateral jumps will challenge you and build multidirectional power. Bilateral jumps provide a solid foundation for these movements and can be supplemented with single-leg hops and alternate-leg bounds as you gain strength and skill.

HIGH-HURDLE JUMP

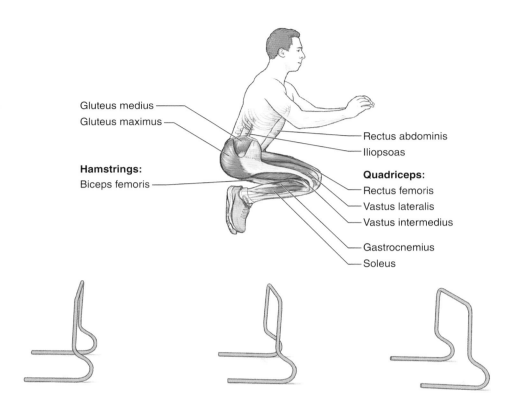

Gluteus medius
Gluteus maximus

Rectus abdominis
Iliopsoas

Hamstrings:
Biceps femoris

Quadriceps:
Rectus femoris
Vastus lateralis
Vastus intermedius

Gastrocnemius
Soleus

Execution

1. High-hurdle jumps require a more significant effort during takeoff, flight, and landing than low-hurdle jumps do. The takeoff must be maximal in effort. Extend powerfully at the hips to attain the appropriate height for flight over the hurdle. Swing the arms upward powerfully to assist in the effort.

2. As you fly over the hurdle, lift the knees, similar to a tuck jump, to ensure adequate clearance over the barrier.

3. Prepare to land by dorsiflexing the feet to ensure a stiff and elastic landing on the balls of the feet. A quick and powerful elastic landing will ensure maximum height on successive jumps.

Muscles Involved

Primary: Gluteus maximus, gluteus medius, quadriceps (rectus femoris, vastus lateralis, vastus intermedius, vastus medialis), soleus, gastrocnemius.

Secondary: Rectus abdominis, iliopsoas, hamstrings (biceps femoris, semi-tendinosus, semimembranosus).

Exercise Notes

High-hurdle jumps are significantly more challenging than most other bilateral jumping exercises because of the need to execute repeated maximal efforts over a fixed barrier. Hurdle heights must be great enough to elicit maximal-effort jumps but not so high that you are at risk of falling and hurting yourself. The combination of performing repeat maximal-height jumps and maintaining short, crisp ground contacts is a complex task that requires significant focus and coordinated muscle recruitment. For this reason, 6 to 10 hurdles in a row will present an adequate challenge in each set without the risk of fatigue. High hurdles also present a psychological barrier and can be intimidating to beginners. Completion of a set of jumps over appropriately selected hurdle heights can build confidence and develop a sense of accomplishment. Monitor ground contacts for each repetition and set to determine optimal volumes of work through the training session.

VARIATION

High-Hurdle Jump With Rotation and Pause Landing

High hurdle jumps can be performed with pause landings to allow you to focus on efficient and stable landing mechanics. The addition of rotational jumps over each hurdle presents a greater challenge through the flight phase and into the landing. Perform the jumps with 90-degree rotations in each direction. Start by facing the hurdle and perform a countermovement to elicit a powerful response in the legs. Initiate the rotation with the arms, shoulders, and head to produce a turning movement over the hurdle. Land in a lateral position on the far side of the hurdle. The second jump starts from a lateral position and finishes with you facing forward for the next repetition. These jumps have a pause between repetitions or can be consecutive elastic jumps depending on your skills and abilities.

LATERAL HURDLE JUMP

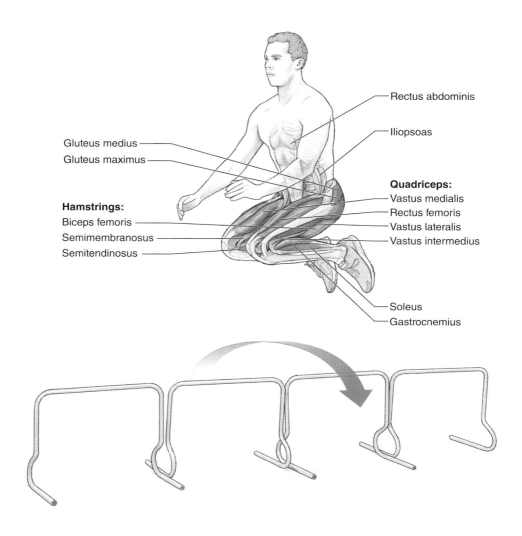

Rectus abdominis

Iliopsoas

Gluteus medius

Gluteus maximus

Quadriceps:
Vastus medialis
Rectus femoris
Vastus lateralis
Vastus intermedius

Hamstrings:
Biceps femoris
Semimembranosus
Semitendinosus

Soleus
Gastrocnemius

Execution

1. Set up a series of hurdles in a line, positioned end to end. Begin by jumping laterally and slightly forward over the first section of hurdles.
2. The lateral jumps will proceed in a zigzag pattern back and forth over the hurdles. Depending on the height of the hurdles, significant hip flexion and knee lift may be required at the top of each jump.
3. Ground contacts for each landing will be short and quick, taking advantage of the elastic response in the feet and lower legs. The arms assist in the execution of each jump, driving forward and up in a rhythmic fashion.

Muscles Involved

Primary: Gluteus maximus, gluteus medius, quadriceps (rectus femoris, vastus lateralis, vastus intermedius, vastus medialis), soleus, gastrocnemius.

Secondary: Rectus abdominis, iliopsoas, hamstrings (biceps femoris, semitendinosus, semimembranosus).

Exercise Notes

You can perform lateral hurdle jumps over low or high hurdles depending on the objectives of the exercise and your abilities. Lower hurdles allow you to focus on tall posture and quick ground contacts. Higher hurdles require greater attention to hip flexion and jump height while also ensuring elastic ground contacts. When implementing lateral hurdle jumps, it is often best to specify the desired number of jumps for each set.

VARIATION

Lateral Hurdle Jump With Medicine Ball Overhead

Using a series of low hurdles arranged in a line, perform lateral jumps back and forth across the barriers while holding a medicine ball directly overhead. This arrangement reinforces tall posture during the jumping movement and also places greater demands on the lower body because the arms do not contribute to the jumping motion.

LOW- AND HIGH-HURDLE JUMP SEQUENCE

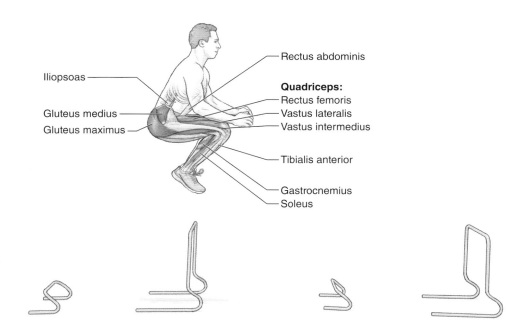

Rectus abdominis

Quadriceps:
Rectus femoris
Vastus lateralis
Vastus intermedius

Iliopsoas

Gluteus medius
Gluteus maximus

Tibialis anterior

Gastrocnemius
Soleus

Execution

1. Start in front of a low hurdle with feet shoulder-width apart. Initiate a double-leg jump over the first hurdle with a modest arm drive.

2. During the flight phase of the first hurdle jump, prepare for an aggressive landing for the second jump in advance of a higher hurdle.

3. Land on the balls of the feet with a quick ground contact in preparation for a powerful takeoff over the high hurdle.

4. Prepare for a soft but quick landing for the preparation of a modest third jump over a lower hurdle.

5. Continue this sequence of alternating-height jumps for 6 to 12 hurdle jumps.

3. On landing, the balls of the feet contact the ground initially, absorbing preliminary forces as the bulk of the weight eventually transfers to the heels. Once heel contact is made, the quadriceps, glutes, and hamstrings assume the bulk of the landing forces in a progressive manner. The torso comes forward as the erector spinae muscles also decelerate the weight of the upper half of the body on landing.

4. The degrees of knee flexion and range of motion covered in the absorption phase depend on the height of the box, your strength, and the specific training objectives for the session.

Muscles Involved

Primary: Gluteus maximus, gluteus medius, quadriceps (rectus femoris, vastus lateralis, vastus intermedius, vastus medialis), hamstrings (biceps femoris, semitendinosus, semimembranosus).

Secondary: Erector spinae (spinalis, longissimus, iliocostalis), soleus, gastrocnemius.

Exercise Notes

Using drop jumps for the specific purpose of training eccentric strength is an effective technique. Acceleration due to gravity can place significant loads on your body in the absence of external weights. Use a lower box to warm up the legs and neuromuscular system. Progress to higher box heights gradually, in the same fashion that a weightlifter would load a barbell through sets of increasingly heavier squats. Use fewer repetitions (3 to 5) with higher box heights, taking into consideration the intensity of the eccentric contractions and the need to recover completely between sets of drop jumps.

VARIATION

Drop Jump Into Split Landing

Perform an alternative bilateral landing from a drop jump in the form of a split landing. This landing places asymmetrical stresses on individual legs, with the partial assistance and support of the other leg. The front leg in the split landing assumes a larger proportion of eccentric load. The rear leg assumes a partial load but plays a larger role in providing support and balance for the landing. Eccentric strength development from these split landings can be helpful in many sports in which athletes are required to perform dynamic lunges.

REACTIVE DEPTH JUMP TO HIGH BOX

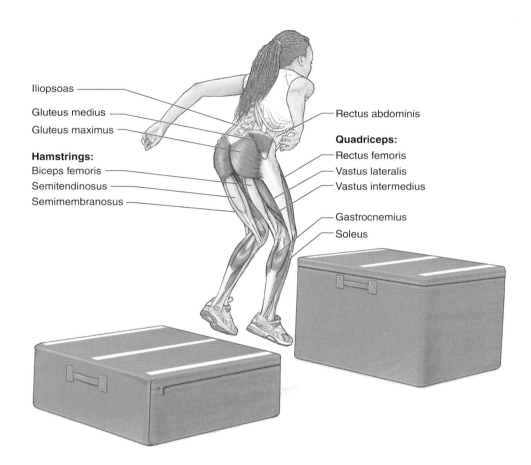

Iliopsoas

Gluteus medius

Gluteus maximus

Hamstrings:

Biceps femoris

Semitendinosus

Semimembranosus

Rectus abdominis

Quadriceps:

Rectus femoris

Vastus lateralis

Vastus intermedius

Gastrocnemius

Soleus

Execution

1. Stand on a low- to moderate-height box. Step off the box and prepare for a simultaneous landing on the ground with both feet.

2. Feet should be dorsiflexed before ground contact to ensure a stiff and elastic landing on the balls of the feet as the action quickly shifts to active plantarflexion.

3. The gathering action of the arms anticipates the takeoff from the ground, timing a strong upward action for the jump onto a high box.

4. Strong hip extension accompanies the dynamic takeoff from the ground, with an emphasis on maximum vertical separation from the ground and, as the knees rise up, a stable, flat-footed landing on the top of the box to finish the repetition.

Muscles Involved

Primary: Gluteus maximus, gluteus medius, quadriceps (rectus femoris, vastus lateralis, vastus intermedius, vastus medialis), soleus, gastrocnemius.

Secondary: Rectus abdominis, iliopsoas, hamstrings (biceps femoris, semi-tendinosus, semimembranosus).

Exercise Notes

Reactive depth jumps onto a high box challenge athletes to maximally recruit the muscles of the lower body to aggressively reverse the direction of the depth jump. The use of gravity to load the lower extremities takes advantage of the elastic properties of the lower legs and feet. This action is accompanied by the strength and power of the quadriceps and gluteal muscles to produce strong extension at the knees and hips. These reactive jumps are one of the most effective means of improving the explosive and reactive properties of the legs and feet, particularly for jumping performance.

As with all depth jumps, the selection of appropriate box heights is critical in determining the success of the exercise. The smaller box must be high enough to adequately load the lower body but not so high as to overload the muscles and tendons and diminish the positive effects of the stretch-shortening cycle. The higher box should be high enough to encourage a significant jump height but not so high that it creates a risk of injury.

VARIATION

Reactive Depth Jump With Rotation

Rotational movements can be incorporated into reactive drop jumps to add a dimension of skill and coordination. Athletes in numerous sporting events and activities are often required to jump and turn, such as a basketball player executing a turnaround jump shot or an American football receiver turning around to make a jumping catch in the end zone. Step off a low box and initiate a 90-degree rotation before landing on the ground. Once you rebound, the next jump can include another 90-degree rotation to land on the top of the high box in the original starting position.

REACTIVE DEPTH JUMP OVER HURDLE

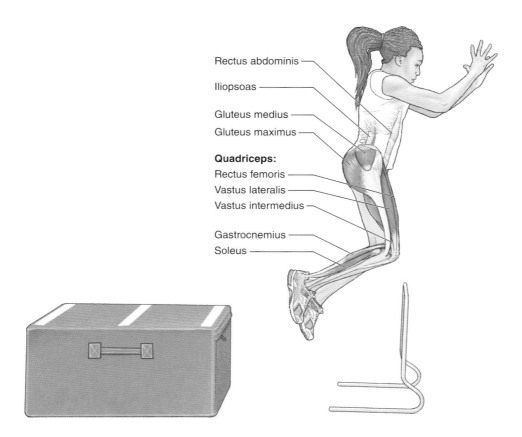

Rectus abdominis

Iliopsoas

Gluteus medius

Gluteus maximus

Quadriceps:

Rectus femoris

Vastus lateralis

Vastus intermedius

Gastrocnemius

Soleus

Execution

1. Stand on a low- to moderate-height box. Step off the box and prepare for a simultaneous landing on the ground with both feet. Feet should be dorsiflexed before ground contact to ensure a rigid and elastic landing on the balls of the feet.

2. Gather the arms in advance of the jump landing, timing a strong upward action of the arms for the jump over a high hurdle.

3. On takeoff, extend the hips powerfully with an emphasis on maximum vertical separation from the ground to attain optimal hip height.

4. Lift the knees to ensure appropriate clearance over the hurdle and land on the far side of the hurdle using the quadriceps and gluteal muscles to decelerate the body.

Muscles Involved

Primary: Gluteus maximus, gluteus medius, quadriceps (rectus femoris, vastus lateralis, vastus intermedius, vastus medialis), soleus, gastrocnemius.

Secondary: Rectus abdominis, iliopsoas.

Exercise Notes

Depth jumps performed with a high hurdle as a vertical barrier not only encourage you to strive for a maximum-height jump but also require you to execute a forceful and stable landing on the other side of the hurdle. This is a good exercise to prepare you for combination jumps involving multiple boxes and hurdles of varying heights arranged in a series. Jumping off boxes and over hurdles can be a fun activity if you view the arrangement of obstacles as a challenge.

VARIATION

Reactive Lateral Depth Jump Over Hurdle

You can perform depth jumps laterally off a low box, landing with both legs simultaneously on the ground to create a reactive lateral takeoff over a moderate-height hurdle. Reactive lateral jumps are useful in developing speed and power for lateral movements required in all types of field and court sports, particularly for reactive defensive movements.

REBOUNDING BOX JUMP

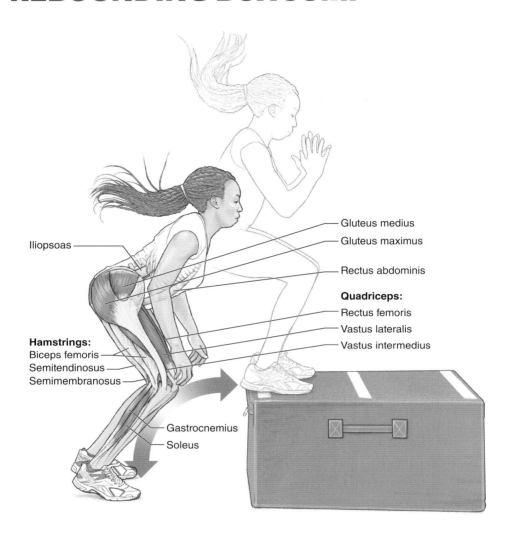

Iliopsoas

Gluteus medius

Gluteus maximus

Rectus abdominis

Quadriceps:
Rectus femoris
Vastus lateralis
Vastus intermedius

Hamstrings:
Biceps femoris
Semitendinosus
Semimembranosus

Gastrocnemius

Soleus

Execution

1. Start with the feet hip-width apart in front of a low- to moderate-height box. Initiate the exercise with a jump onto the top of the box, lightly contacting the surface with the balls of the feet and rebounding back off the box.

2. On the descent backward to the ground, prepare to land on the balls of the feet and react quickly off the ground with another jump forward up to the top of the same box.

3. Continue jumping back and forth from the top of the box to the ground in a rhythmic fashion, with quick, elastic foot contacts on both ends of the exercise.

4. Arm action during the jumps cover a short range of motion, timed with the impulse of each jumping effort.

Muscles Involved

Primary: Gluteus maximus, gluteus medius, quadriceps (rectus femoris, vastus lateralis, vastus intermedius, vastus medialis), soleus, gastrocnemius.

Secondary: Rectus abdominis, iliopsoas, hamstrings (biceps femoris, semi-tendinosus, semimembranosus).

Exercise Notes

In rebounding box jumps, you use a low- to moderate-height box and execute repetitive elastic jumps back and forth. The jump back onto the ground creates a greater posterior emphasis on the landing because many forward jumps place more eccentric stress on anterior structures such as the quadriceps and knee tendons. The objective is to maintain quick, elastic foot contacts on both the ground and the top of the box through each set of jumps in a rhythmic fashion. If you are spending too much time on the ground, use a lower box. Jumps can be implemented in sets of 6 to 12 repetitions, depending on the height of the box.

VARIATION

Rebounding Jump With Single-Leg Landing

The foot contacts on the ground will be of greater force than the landings on the top of the box during rebounding jumps. To create a more complex exercise, contact the top of the box with a single-leg landing, where impact forces are much less, while still maintaining double-foot landings on the ground. The single-leg touches can alternate between the right and left foot throughout the set.

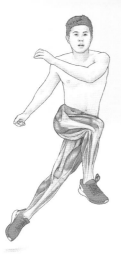

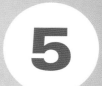
5

UNILATERAL LOWER-BODY EXERCISES

Bilateral lower-body plyometrics provide a good foundation of exercises for developing strength, power, and elasticity in the legs and feet. Unilateral jumps add a specific element to a plyometric program that can also place greater loads on individual legs. Single-leg plyometrics may be considered a more complex means of training the lower body, requiring greater coordination, balance, and body awareness. However, some athletes may find that single-leg exercises are easier to incorporate into their training programs because they may be more like the natural movement patterns found in their sports.

You can use unilateral plyometric exercises early in a training program provided that you emphasize technical proficiency and follow a gradual progression of work. Initially, you can perform submaximal versions of unilateral jumps with more forceful bilateral exercises to ensure that you have adequate exposure to all types of plyometric exercises. Both types of movements can be beneficial to the development of strength, power, and speed when introduced in the correct sequence and appropriate volumes. Overreliance on bilateral exercises only may leave a gap in specific skill development for explosive sporting movements, while excessive unilateral work can lead to overuse injuries, particularly in the area of the sacroiliac joint and hips.

Unilateral plyometric exercises can be useful in developing single-leg power and elasticity required for sprinting and jumping movements in various sports. You can integrate various exercises into a training program to improve single-leg landing techniques and abilities as well as prepare for the demands of hard-cutting movements and direction changes. Single-leg exercises place significantly greater demands on hip, knee, and ankle control than double-leg exercises do. Once a foundation of strength and power is developed through the use of bilateral plyometric exercises and other supportive strength training methods, the addition of single-leg exercises can help to refine specific movement skills and improve overall power delivery through individual legs.

CONCENTRIC BOX JUMPS

Jumping up onto a box is a simple way to develop explosive power abilities while minimizing landing forces. The box should be high enough to elicit a powerful jump but not too high to put your safety in jeopardy. Pure concentric box jumps with a single leg are even more challenging than double-leg jumps. You must produce enough power with a single leg to propel yourself safely up onto the top of a box. Improvements in unilateral power from concentric box jumps can help to develop single-leg jumping abilities for sports such as basketball as well as starting strength and power for sprinting abilities.

BOUNDING

Basic alternate-leg bounding is a foundational exercise for developing unilateral power for speed training. The adaptations created through bounding increase stride length and overall hip extension power for single-leg jumps. You can incorporate bounding variations into a training program to develop specific characteristics that improve performance and overall athleticism. Distances of 20 to 40 meters are commonly used for bounding sets, depending on individual circumstances. Include adequate recovery between sets to preserve the quality of work through a training session.

SINGLE-LEG HOPS

Single-leg hops are effective in developing leg strength and power in individual legs. Single-leg hopping combines the strong downward force capabilities of the hopping leg with a dynamic knee drive of the swinging leg. The precise timing and coordination of both movements ultimately determine the distance and velocity of each hop. Ensure that you properly manage hopping volume to avoid overuse injuries. You should perform distance hopping for no more than 30 meters to maintain the quality of performance in individual sets.

HOPPING AND BOUNDING COMBINATIONS

Combining hops and bounds in a single set of jumps is a good way to improve overall coordination and athleticism as well as evenly distribute the number of ground contacts over both legs. While hopping on one leg can be very effective in developing strength and power in that individual limb, it can also be very stressful to carry out continuous hops over numerous sets. Alternating hopping and bounding diffuses leg stresses while still accumulating the benefits of unilateral work over time.

Because hopping and bounding combinations can be difficult for beginners to learn, keep the patterns simple and submaximal at first. Start with simple ankle hops and bounds to build rhythm and skill. As you improve at a given pattern, place greater effort on the distance of individual hops and bounds as well as the overall speed of execution. The use of cones along the field can help determine the spacing of jumps as well as the leg involved.

SINGLE-LEG BOX HOP FROM LUNGE

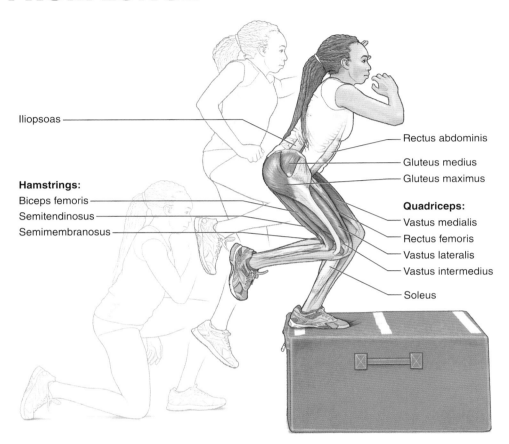

Iliopsoas

Rectus abdominis

Gluteus medius

Gluteus maximus

Hamstrings:
Biceps femoris
Semitendinosus
Semimembranosus

Quadriceps:
Vastus medialis
Rectus femoris
Vastus lateralis
Vastus intermedius

Soleus

Execution

1. Start in a lunge position with one leg in front of the body with the knee at 90 degrees flexion and the opposite leg trailing behind the body with the knee on the floor to provide stability. Set the arms in opposition to the legs to gather in preparation for the upward drive on takeoff.

2. Initiate the movement with the arms, simultaneously emphasizing a strong vertical push downward with the front foot and a strong knee drive upward with the rear leg.

3. After the powerful knee drive from the free-swinging leg, perform a leg exchange to allow the initial front leg to land upon the top of the box, softly absorbing the force of the landing.

Muscles Involved

Primary: Gluteus maximus, gluteus medius, quadriceps (rectus femoris, vastus lateralis, vastus intermedius, vastus medialis), hamstrings (biceps femoris, semitendinosus, semimembranosus).

Secondary: Rectus abdominis, iliopsoas, soleus.

Exercise Notes

Single-leg box hops from a lunge position are an advanced exercise for development of unilateral power. The low starting position requires greater involvement from the hamstrings and gluteal muscles of the front takeoff leg. A strong knee drive from the rear leg also helps to vault you powerfully to the top of the box. A low- to moderate-height box is recommended for initial sessions to ensure safe landings. As abilities improve, a higher box will encourage greater performances. Having the takeoff leg also be the landing leg requires more coordination and makes the jump more challenging. A single-arm drive working in opposition to the lower body helps to provide upward propulsion but also counterbalances the torque created by the single-leg effort.

VARIATION

Standing Single-Leg Box Hop

Performing single-leg box hops from a standing position allows for quicker takeoff. The higher hip position also permits jumping onto a higher box, even though the range of motion of the takeoff is reduced as compared with a start from the lunge position. You also can incorporate a strong countermovement in the standing position or even a single step into the takeoff. These exercises add a single-leg hop before the jump to the top of the box, adding more profound elastic response to the takeoff.

ANKLE BOUND

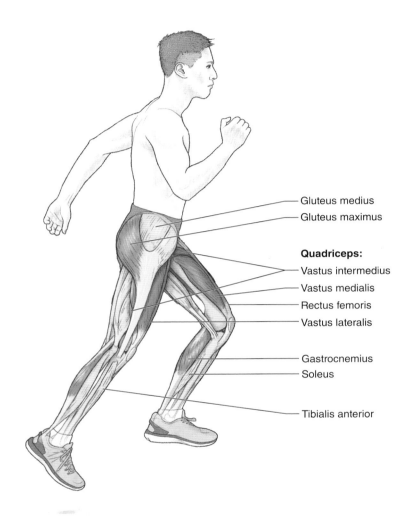

Gluteus medius
Gluteus maximus

Quadriceps:
Vastus intermedius
Vastus medialis
Rectus femoris
Vastus lateralis

Gastrocnemius
Soleus

Tibialis anterior

Execution

1. Stand with the feet hip-width apart. Initiate the first bound by driving the knee and the opposite arm forward. The knee drive will be moderate in height as the intent is not to bound as far as possible, but set up a quick and elastic landing.

2. Prepare for landing by dorsiflexing the foot on ground preparation to add pre-tension in the muscles of the calf.

3. Land the bound with minimal knee flexion on ground contact, aiming for a midfoot ground contact and a tall posture on landing.

4. Drive the knee of the free leg forward to initiate the second bound and continue with this cyclical bounding movement for 10 to 20 meters.

Muscles Involved

Primary: Gluteus maximus, quadriceps (rectus femoris, vastus lateralis, vastus intermedius, vastus medialis), gastrocnemius.

Secondary: Gluteus medius, soleus, tibialis anterior.

Exercise Notes

Shorter-length bounding exercises that focus on the elastic properties of the lower legs and feet are known as ankle bounds. Athletes rely less on knee drive and powerful hip extension in this exercise and more on the action of the feet. Ground preparation for individual takeoffs includes active dorsiflexion of the feet to enhance stiffness of the ankle joint on landings. Quick and sharp ground contacts create both height and length on each bound, landing with a midfoot stance. Arm action should also be quick and short in range to match the action of the lower body.

VARIATION

Lateral Ankle Bound

You can introduce a slight side-to-side motion on the ankle bounds to simulate foot contacts during lateral agility movements. The lateral deviations on the bounds will improve overall ankle strengthening as well as reinforce optimal hip and knee control on ground contact.

STRAIGHT-LEG BOUND

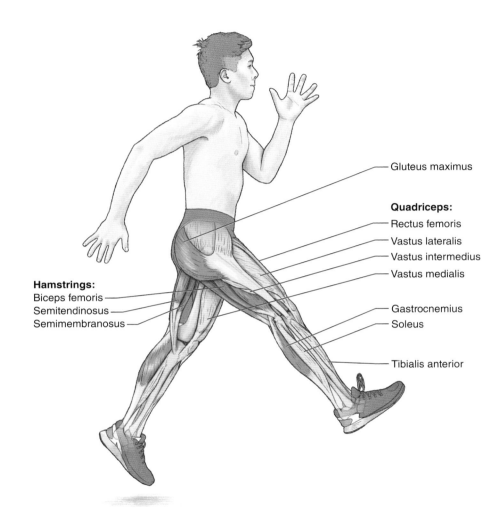

Gluteus maximus

Quadriceps:
Rectus femoris
Vastus lateralis
Vastus intermedius
Vastus medialis

Gastrocnemius
Soleus

Tibialis anterior

Hamstrings:
Biceps femoris
Semitendinosus
Semimembranosus

Execution

1. Stand with feet hip-width apart. Initiate the first bound by sweeping the lead leg forward with the knee joint fully extended. The opposite arm sweeps forward to match the range of the lead leg.

2. Quickly draw the lead leg back toward the ground with the foot dorsiflexed to prepare for a dynamic landing.

3. Aim for a midfoot ground contact and a tall posture on landing with minimal knee flexion.

4. Drive the knee of the free leg forward to initiate the second straight-leg bound and continue with this cyclical bounding movement for 10 to 20 meters.

Muscles Involved

Primary: Gluteus maximus, gastrocnemius, hamstrings (biceps femoris, semitendinosus, semimembranosus).

Secondary: Quadriceps (rectus femoris, vastus lateralis, vastus intermedius, vastus medialis), soleus, tibialis anterior.

Exercise Notes

Bounding performed with limited knee flexion and the downward sweeping motion of the legs relies on elasticity in the lower legs and feet as well as significant hamstring strength. Straight-leg bounding teaches you to recruit the hamstrings as powerful hip extensors for propulsion in sprinting and jumping movements. The arms swing in an extended fashion to match the rhythm and action of the lower body.

SPEED BOUND

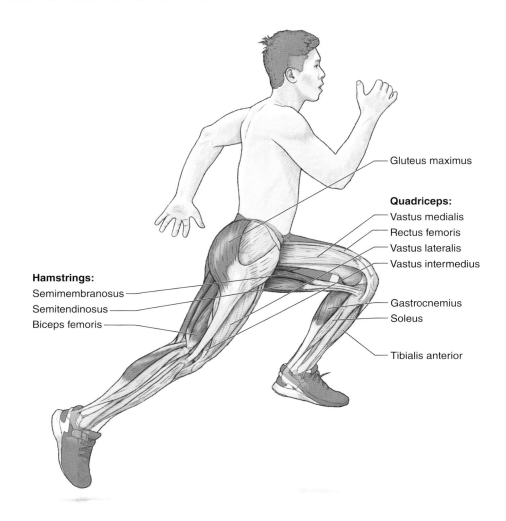

Gluteus maximus

Quadriceps:
Vastus medialis
Rectus femoris
Vastus lateralis
Vastus intermedius

Gastrocnemius
Soleus

Tibialis anterior

Hamstrings:
Semimembranosus
Semitendinosus
Biceps femoris

Execution

1. Stand with feet hip-width apart. Initiate first bound by driving the knee of the lead leg forward at a relatively flat trajectory. The opposite arm sweeps forward to match the range of the lead leg.

2. Quickly draw the lead leg back toward the ground with the foot dorsiflexed to prepare for a dynamic landing a few inches in front of the center of mass.

3. Aim for a midfoot ground contact and a tall posture on landing with minimal knee flexion.

4. Quickly drive the knee of the free leg forward to initiate the second bound and continue with this cyclical bounding movement for 20 to 30 meters in distance.

Muscles Involved

Primary: Gluteus maximus, gastrocnemius, hamstrings (biceps femoris, semitendinosus, semimembranosus).

Secondary: Quadriceps (rectus femoris, vastus lateralis, vastus intermedius, vastus medialis), soleus, tibialis anterior.

Exercise Notes

Bounding for speed will more closely resemble the action of a sprint stride. The trajectory of the bounds will be relatively flat with a greater emphasis on horizontal acceleration and velocity. The stride of speed bounds is exaggerated compared with a regular running stride, with a greater knee drive on each step and greater extension at the hip. Arm action in a speed bound matches the range and speed of the legs.

UPHILL BOUND

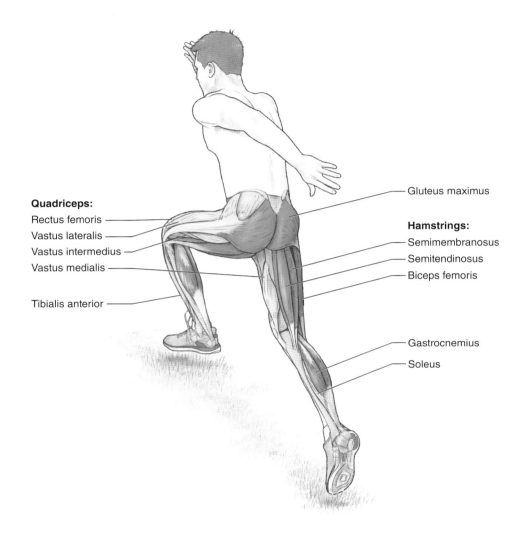

Quadriceps:
Rectus femoris
Vastus lateralis
Vastus intermedius
Vastus medialis

Tibialis anterior

Gluteus maximus

Hamstrings:
Semimembranosus
Semitendinosus
Biceps femoris

Gastrocnemius
Soleus

Execution

1. Stand with feet hip-width apart at the bottom of a gradual hill or incline. Initiate first bound by driving the knee of the lead leg forward to accelerate up the hill. The opposite arm sweeps forward to match the range of the lead leg.

2. Quickly draw the lead leg back toward the ground with the foot dorsiflexed to prepare for a dynamic landing a few inches in front of the body.

3. Aim for a midfoot ground contact and drive the body forward with a powerful hip extension motion.

4. Quickly drive the knee of the free leg forward to initiate the second bound and continue with this cyclical bounding movement uphill for 20 to 30 meters.

Muscles Involved

Primary: Gluteus maximus, gastrocnemius, hamstrings (biceps femoris, semitendinosus, semimembranosus).

Secondary: Quadriceps (rectus femoris, vastus lateralis, vastus intermedius, vastus medialis), soleus, tibialis anterior.

Exercise Notes

Bounding uphill is a useful means of teaching bounding and enhances hip extension during bounding, jumping, and sprinting. Uphill bounding is also less stressful on the body than similar bounds on flat ground. The landing forces are reduced in an uphill scenario and provide an easier condition under which to learn the skill of bounding. It is important to select an uphill surface that is not slick or uneven, minimizing the chance of slipping while executing the bounding steps.

VARIATION

Lateral Uphill Bound

You can perform uphill bounds with a slight side-to-side motion to add a lateral dimension to the exercise. The combination of powering up the hill and introducing a lateral push can simulate the acceleration requirements for ice hockey and speed skating as well as agility movements in field sports.

CROSSOVER BOUND

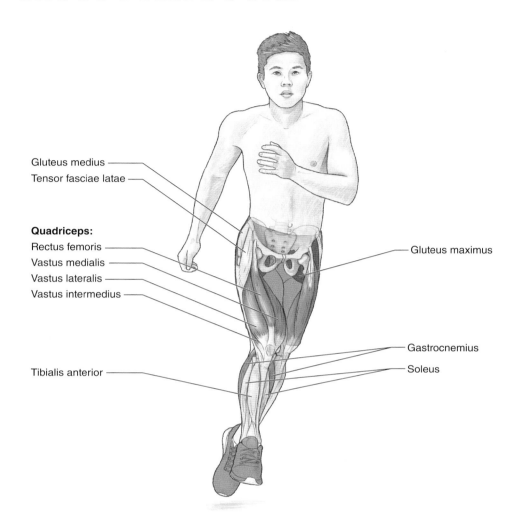

Gluteus medius
Tensor fasciae latae

Quadriceps:
Rectus femoris
Vastus medialis
Vastus lateralis
Vastus intermedius

Tibialis anterior

Gluteus maximus

Gastrocnemius
Soleus

Execution

1. Stand with feet hip-width apart. Initiate first bound by driving the knee of the lead leg forward and across the midline of the body. The opposite arm sweeps forward and across the midline of the body to match the range of the lead leg.

2. The flight phase of the bound should be relatively short with an emphasis on quality of ground contact as opposed to bounding distance.

3. As the lead leg descends toward the ground, prepare for ground contact with the foot dorsiflexed and execute a firm but quick midfoot landing.

4. Quickly drive the knee of the free leg forward and across the midline of the body to initiate the second lateral crossover bound. Repeat this motion over 10 to 20 meters.

Muscles Involved

Primary: Gluteus maximus, gastrocnemius, quadriceps (rectus femoris, vastus lateralis, vastus intermedius, vastus medialis).

Secondary: Gluteus medius, soleus, tibialis anterior, tensor fasciae latae.

Exercise Notes

While lateral bounds can provide additional training of muscles on the lateral portions of the lower extremities, bounds that involve the legs crossing over the midline of the body place additional demands on the medial areas of the legs. This bounding exercise can simulate the mechanics and forces experienced during change of direction and cutting movements in many team sports such as soccer, basketball, American football, lacrosse, and rugby. Stepping across the midline of the body to turn or change direction can place significant stresses on a single leg. You should introduce crossover bounding at submaximal intensities and over shorter distances initially to strengthen the required muscles and develop specific coordination. It is also important to execute these bounds on a training surface that is even and firm.

CARIOCA BOUND

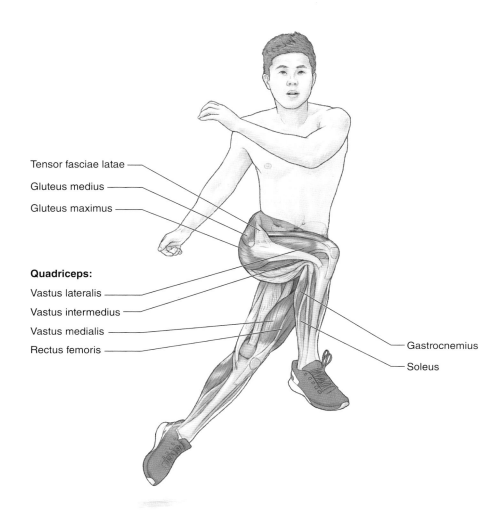

Tensor fasciae latae

Gluteus medius

Gluteus maximus

Quadriceps:

Vastus lateralis

Vastus intermedius

Vastus medialis

Rectus femoris

Gastrocnemius

Soleus

Execution

1. Stand lateral to the direction of travel. Initiate first bound by driving the knee of the far leg across the body for maximum distance.

2. On landing, push laterally to accelerate the body sideways and attain distance on the next stride. Swing the arms in opposition to the legs to maintain balance and generate greater lateral power.

3. Step behind the body on the next lateral stride. This stride will be of significantly less distance but will maintain the momentum of the lateral motion.

4. Continue to bound across the body with both a stride in front and then a stride behind the body to accelerate over a distance of 10 to 30 meters.

Muscles Involved

Primary: Gluteus maximus, gluteus medius, gastrocnemius, quadriceps (rectus femoris, vastus lateralis, vastus intermedius, vastus medialis).

Secondary: Soleus, tensor fasciae latae, adductors (longus, magnus, brevis).

Exercise Notes

This exercise incorporates an elongated stride pattern in the regular carioca drill by stepping across the body to provide lateral propulsion. In one stride you step across the front of the body to generate downward force and horizontal propulsion. The next stride steps in behind the body to provide the same lateral propulsion. The stepping across and behind the body by strides creates rotational forces between the hips and shoulders because the arms counterrotate in relation to power produced by the legs. The range of motion by extremities covered in carioca bounding is much more significant than in the regular exercise because you cover more horizontal distance in each stride.

HURDLE BOUND

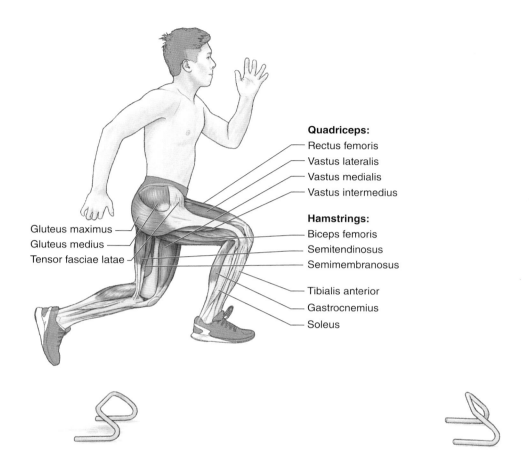

Quadriceps:
Rectus femoris
Vastus lateralis
Vastus medialis
Vastus intermedius

Hamstrings:
Biceps femoris
Semitendinosus
Semimembranosus

Tibialis anterior
Gastrocnemius
Soleus

Gluteus maximus
Gluteus medius
Tensor fasciae latae

Execution

1. Stand a few meters behind a row of low hurdles. Jog toward the hurdles and begin with a single bound over the first hurdle.

2. During the flight phase over the hurdle, prepare for ground contact with slight dorsiflexion of the front foot.

3. Contact the ground with a midfoot landing and drive the opposite knee forward and up to initiate the second hurdle bound. Arms drive in opposition to the legs to counterbalance the body.

4. Continue to perform alternate-leg bounds over the series of hurdles in a rhythmic fashion, focusing on short ground contact times and a strong knee drive.

5. Perform bounds over 6 to 12 evenly spaced hurdles.

Muscles Involved

Primary: Gluteus maximus, gluteus medius, gastrocnemius, quadriceps (rectus femoris, vastus lateralis, vastus intermedius, vastus medialis), hamstrings (biceps femoris, semitendinosus, semimembranosus).

Secondary: Soleus, tensor fasciae latae, tibialis anterior.

Exercise Notes

Hurdles can provide greater vertical deflection on individual bounds. The hurdles need not be very high to provide a significant difference in height as compared with regular bounding. In some cases, hurdles of 6 to 10 inches can provide a significant difference to bounding flight paths. Spacing of the hurdles should match your bounding abilities to ensure that you do not deviate too far from your regular stride lengths and rhythm. At most, 12 hurdles should be used in bounding sets to ensure that the quality of bounding mechanics is maintained.

VARIATION

Lateral Bound Over Hurdles

Low hurdles can be arranged in a continuous line to encourage you to bound back and forth across the line of hurdles as you move forward. The lateral bounds need not be wide. The hurdles can provide additional incentive for gaining vertical height on your bounds while encouraging a lateral aspect to the exercise.

ANKLE HOP

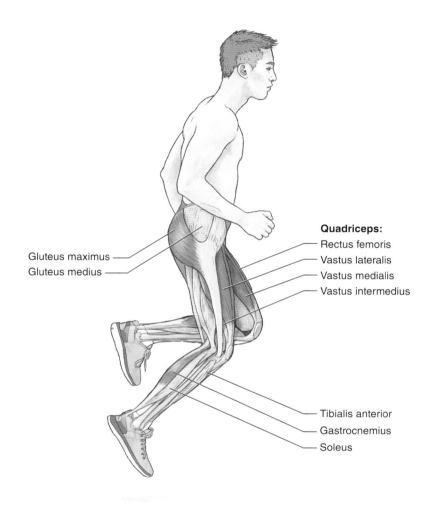

Gluteus maximus

Gluteus medius

Quadriceps:
Rectus femoris
Vastus lateralis
Vastus medialis
Vastus intermedius

Tibialis anterior
Gastrocnemius
Soleus

Execution

1. Stand with feet hip-width apart. Initiate the first single-leg hop by driving the opposite knee forward. The knee drive will be moderate in height because the intent is not to hop as far as possible but to set up a quick and elastic landing for each hop.

2. Prepare for landing with the same hopping leg by dorsiflexing the foot during ground preparation to add pre-tension to the muscles of the calf.

3. Land each single-leg hop with minimal knee flexion on ground contact, aiming for a midfoot ground contact and a tall posture on landing.

4. Perform continuous hops on the same leg in this fashion for 10 to 20 meters. Arms will drive in opposition to the legs to counterbalance the action of the lower extremities. Switch legs.

Muscles Involved

Primary: Gluteus maximus, quadriceps (rectus femoris, vastus lateralis, vastus intermedius, vastus medialis), gastrocnemius.

Secondary: Gluteus medius, soleus, tibialis anterior.

Exercise Notes

Short-range hops with limited knee flexion on ground contact enhance the contribution of the feet and lower legs to the hopping motion. Active ground contacts are imperative, reinforcing the need for stiffness in all of the joints of the lower body, producing elasticity from connective tissues. The ankle hops will be of short distance, with arm action mirroring the rhythm and range of the lower body.

POWER HOP

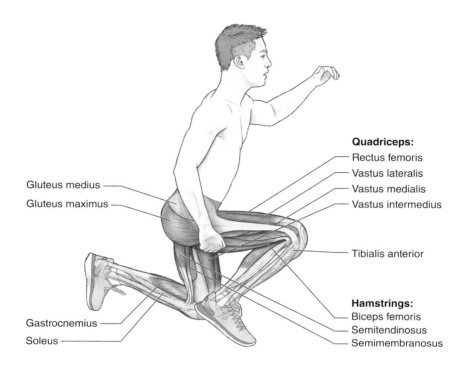

Quadriceps:
Rectus femoris
Vastus lateralis
Vastus medialis
Vastus intermedius

Gluteus medius
Gluteus maximus

Tibialis anterior

Hamstrings:
Biceps femoris
Semitendinosus
Semimembranosus

Gastrocnemius
Soleus

Execution

1. Stand with feet hip-width apart. Initiate the first single-leg hop by power-fully driving the opposite knee forward. The knee drives to the height of the hip in order to provide maximum height and distance on each hop.

2. After pushing off the ground, the knee of the hopping leg cycles forward to prepare for the next jump.

3. Prepare for landing with the hopping leg by dorsiflexing the foot as it sweeps downward to add pre-tension to the muscles of the lower leg and foot.

4. On landing, focus on contacting the ground with a midfoot stance for stability and rigidity.

5. Perform continuous powerful hops on the same leg in this fashion for 10 to 20 meters. Arms drive in opposition to the legs to counterbalance the action of the lower extremities. Switch legs.

Muscles Involved

Primary: Gluteus maximus, quadriceps (rectus femoris, vastus lateralis, vastus intermedius, vastus medialis), gastrocnemius, hamstrings (biceps femoris, semitendinosus, semimembranosus).

Secondary: Gluteus medius, soleus, tibialis anterior.

Exercise Notes

You can introduce hops of greater distance to develop strength and power in all of the muscles of the legs. Emphasis on vertical force production will yield improvements in both the distance and height of single-leg hops. Greater recruitment of the quadriceps, hamstrings, and glutes will be involved in power hops, particularly as you gain velocity and distance over the execution of the exercise.

VARIATION

Speed Hops

By shifting the emphasis from distance of individual hops to speed of movement, you can develop greater single-leg speed and power abilities through the use of speed hops. The height of these hops will be much lower than those achieved in power hops with a flatter trajectory for each hop. Increase the frequency of the hops and focus on accelerating with each successive hop.

REVERSE HOP

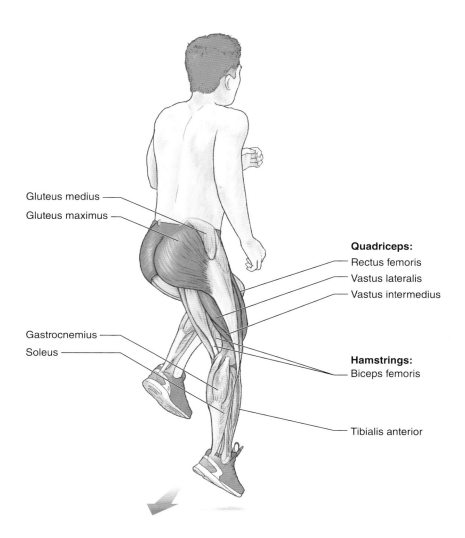

Gluteus medius

Gluteus maximus

Gastrocnemius

Soleus

Quadriceps:
Rectus femoris
Vastus lateralis
Vastus intermedius

Hamstrings:
Biceps femoris

Tibialis anterior

Execution

1. Stand with feet hip-width apart and your back facing the direction of travel.

2. Initiate the first single-leg hop by pushing on the ground with the hopping leg to drive the body backward. The free swinging leg oscillates back and forth in opposition to the hopping leg.

3. After the initial push-off, the hopping leg will reach back for the second hop, landing on the ball of the foot.

4. Ground contacts should be quick and light to prevent losses in momentum.

5. Perform continuous reverse hops on the same leg in this fashion for 10 to 20 meters. Arms drive in opposition to the legs to counterbalance the action of the lower extremities. Switch legs.

Muscles Involved

Primary: Quadriceps (rectus femoris, vastus lateralis, vastus intermedius, vastus medialis), gastrocnemius, gluteus maximus.

Secondary: Gluteus medius, soleus, tibialis anterior, hamstrings (biceps femoris, semitendinosus, semimembranosus).

Exercise Notes

Hopping backward on one leg can build quadriceps strength but also assist with multidirectional movement abilities. Many sports require some degree of back-pedaling, particularly in a defensive scenario. Reverse hopping can strengthen the muscles required for all types of backward movements. Sets of reverse hops can be implemented for distances of 10 to 20 meters, depending on your strength, abilities, and experience.

LATERAL ABDUCTING HOP

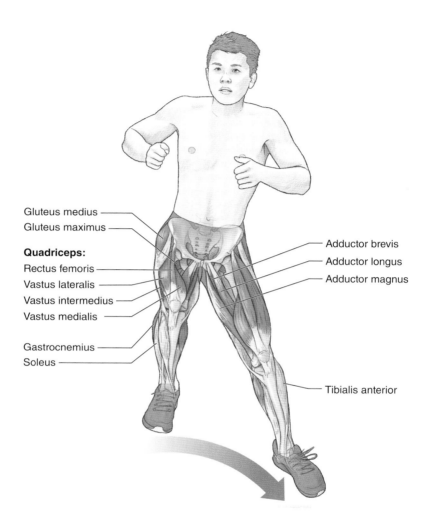

Gluteus medius

Gluteus maximus

Quadriceps:

Rectus femoris

Vastus lateralis

Vastus intermedius

Vastus medialis

Gastrocnemius

Soleus

Adductor brevis

Adductor longus

Adductor magnus

Tibialis anterior

Execution

1. Stand with the feet hip-width apart and facing laterally to the direction of travel.

2. Initiate the first lateral hop by pushing outward (abduction) with the far leg to drive the body sideways. The free-swinging leg abducts from the other side of the body to counterbalance the action of the hopping leg.

3. After the initial lateral push-off, the hopping leg reaches across the body to land the second hop, and the ground contact occurs at the midfoot position.

4. Ground contacts should be quick and light to prevent losses in momentum, minimizing any reaching or excessive pushing efforts.

5. Perform continuous lateral hops on the same leg in this fashion for 5 to 10 meters. Switch legs.

Muscles Involved

Primary: Quadriceps (rectus femoris, vastus lateralis, vastus intermedius, vastus medialis), gastrocnemius, gluteus medius, adductors (longus, magnus, brevis).

Secondary: Gluteus maximus, soleus, tibialis anterior.

Exercise Notes

Hopping laterally on a single leg can strengthen the lower extremities for cutting and change-of-direction movements required in various sports. Not only will lateral hops strengthen the muscles around the ankles, knees, and hips for performance and injury prevention, but these exercises help develop fine motor skills for specific movement patterns required in sport. You need to cover only short distances in lateral hopping exercises (no more than 5 to 10 meters).

VARIATION

Lateral Adducting Hop

Perform lateral hops equally with both abduction and adduction movements to balance the contribution of muscles on either side of the hip, knee, and ankle joints. The adduction motion is carried out by the leg closest to the direction of travel. The push across the body should be quick to allow the leg to recover back to a safe landing position for successive hops.

TWO HOPS PLUS ONE BOUND

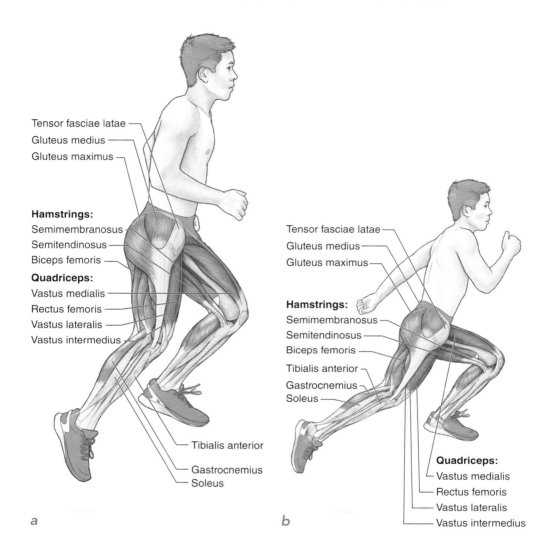

Tensor fasciae latae
Gluteus medius
Gluteus maximus

Hamstrings:
Semimembranosus
Semitendinosus
Biceps femoris
Quadriceps:
Vastus medialis
Rectus femoris
Vastus lateralis
Vastus intermedius

Tibialis anterior
Gastrocnemius
Soleus

a

Tensor fasciae latae
Gluteus medius
Gluteus maximus

Hamstrings:
Semimembranosus
Semitendinosus
Biceps femoris
Tibialis anterior
Gastrocnemius
Soleus

Quadriceps:
Vastus medialis
Rectus femoris
Vastus lateralis
Vastus intermedius

b

Execution

1. Stand with the feet hip-width apart. Initiate the first single-leg hop by driving the opposite knee forward. The knee drive is moderate in height because the intent is to generate moderate-length hops to combine with bounds.

2. After two successive hops, transition into a bound onto the other leg. Dorsiflex the foot for ground preparation on both hopping and bounding landings. Initiate two more hops with the landing leg.

3. Land each single-leg hop and bound with minimal knee flexion on ground contact, aiming for a midfoot ground contact and a tall posture on landing.

4. Perform the continuous cycle of two hops and one bound for 15 to 30 meters. Arms drive in opposition to the legs to counterbalance the action of the lower extremities. Switch legs.

Muscles Involved

Primary: Gluteus maximus, gluteus medius, gastrocnemius, quadriceps (rectus femoris, vastus lateralis, vastus intermedius, vastus medialis), hamstrings (biceps femoris, semitendinosus, semimembranosus).

Secondary: Soleus, tensor fasciae latae, tibialis anterior.

Exercise Notes

One of the most basic combination drills is performing two hops and one bound alternately. The single bound is a transition between the two hops on each leg. Two hops on the right leg switch into a single bound to the left leg, where two more hops are added. The exchange occurs throughout the drill with each leg handling the same amount of ground contacts. When implementing this drill, identify the total number of cycles through each pattern that you desire. Hopping and bounding to a specific distance may yield different results for each set; one leg puts in significantly more work than another over the entirety of the training session.

VARIATION

Three Hops and Three Bounds

The addition of more hops and bounds introduces a higher degree of complexity to a combination exercise; an odd number of bounds always places you onto the other leg for hops. The inclusion of more bounds also creates the potential for higher horizontal velocities within the exercise. Transitioning from bounds to hops challenges you to maintain higher velocities and, in most cases, higher force production in the hopping leg. If you learn to handle high horizontal velocities in both bounds and hops, you will be able to generate enough for both fast accelerations and decelerations.

MULTIDIRECTIONAL HOP

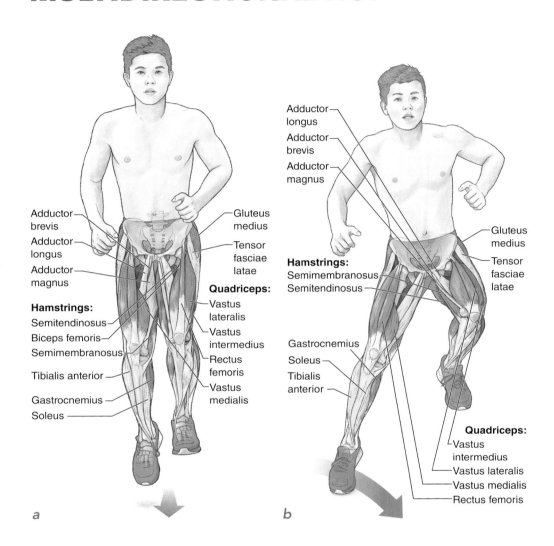

Adductor brevis
Adductor longus
Adductor magnus

Hamstrings:
Semitendinosus
Biceps femoris
Semimembranosus

Tibialis anterior
Gastrocnemius
Soleus

Gluteus medius
Tensor fasciae latae

Quadriceps:
Vastus lateralis
Vastus intermedius
Rectus femoris
Vastus medialis

Adductor longus
Adductor brevis
Adductor magnus

Hamstrings:
Semimembranosus
Semitendinosus

Gastrocnemius
Soleus
Tibialis anterior

Gluteus medius
Tensor fasciae latae

Quadriceps:
Vastus intermedius
Vastus lateralis
Vastus medialis
Rectus femoris

a

b

Execution

1. Stand with the feet hip-width apart. Initiate the first single-leg hop by driving the opposite knee forward. The knee drive is moderate in height because the intent is to generate short- to moderate-length forward hops to combine with lateral hops.

2. Dorsiflex the foot for ground preparation on all hopping landings to ensure quick and powerful ground contacts.

3. After two successive forward hops, transition into a lateral abducting hop (pushing outward) to change direction.

4. Continue forward with two more hops and then change direction with a lateral adducting hop.

5. Land each single-leg hop and bound with minimal knee flexion on ground contact, aiming for a midfoot ground contact and a tall posture on landing.

6. Perform the continuous cycle of two hops and one lateral hop for 10 to 15 meters. Switch hopping legs after each set. Arms drive in opposition to the legs to counterbalance the action of the lower extremities.

Muscles Involved

Primary: Gluteus maximus, gluteus medius, gastrocnemius, quadriceps (rectus femoris, vastus lateralis, vastus intermedius, vastus medialis), hamstrings (biceps femoris, semitendinosus, semimembranosus).

Secondary: Soleus, tensor fasciae latae, tibialis anterior, adductors (brevis, magnus, longus).

Exercise Notes

A more complex series of hopping exercises that you can introduce as a multisport athlete are multidirectional hopping movements. You can do these exercises in place, over distance, or through a series of markings on a gym floor or field. The objective is to incorporate a combination of quick and precise forward and lateral hops into the routines. Draw or tape lines on a floor or field to identify lines that you can jump back and forth across for the purpose of training single-leg speed and agility. Ensure that different movements (forward and lateral) and both legs are equally implemented to prevent overuse.

VARIATION

Forward and Backward Hopping and Bounding Combinations

Exercises that focus on deceleration and change of direction include hopping movements that incorporate forward and backward jumps. A common approach is to perform two or three hops forward followed by a hop backward. You would then bound onto the opposite leg and repeat the hopping pattern. This pattern could alternate over five or six cycles of the pattern. Keep the forward hops moderate in length to allow the change of direction backward to be feasible. If too much forward momentum is generated on a single-leg hop, it is virtually impossible to reverse the direction of the hop, regardless of your strength. You can then modify these exercises to include lateral hops and bounds so that you cover all directions of movement in these drills.

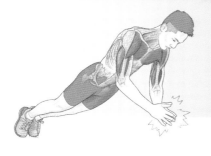

6

UPPER-BODY EXERCISES

Plyometric exercises targeting the upper body can be useful in developing overall strength, power, and speed for all types of sporting movements involving the arms. Dynamic movements, involving pushing and pulling actions by the arms, benefit from activating the stretch-shortening cycle and taking advantage of the elastic properties of upper-body muscles and connective tissues. Explosive and elastic training activities of the upper body improve not only alactic abilities but also the economy of longer-duration aerobic activities performed by the upper extremities. The comprehensive benefits of an effective upper-body plyometric program extend well beyond the realm of explosive qualities.

Upper-body plyometric exercises must follow a gradual progression of work to maintain the health and performance capabilities of the upper extremities. Because of the complex anatomy of the shoulder, you must carefully plan the process of loading the upper body with dynamic movements, emphasizing executing each exercise with optimal biomechanics. Exercise selection must be appropriate for the sport in question but also ensure health and safety. As with any explosive or high-speed exercise, take time to integrate both the skill requirements and the physiological demands of upper-body plyometrics before assuming heavy training loads.

Figure 6.1 details the upper-body muscles involved in athletic movements. Explosive plyometric pushing movements receive significant contributions from the pectoralis major, anterior deltoids, and triceps brachii. Powerful pulling movements in a plyometric program are greatly supported by the biceps brachii, trapezius, and latissimus dorsi. Numerous other upper-body muscles play a supporting role in providing structural stability and precision of movement for athletic skills. Along with supporting illustrations, the movements of the muscles are detailed for each of the prescribed upper-body plyometric exercises.

A majority of the plyometric exercises in this chapter involve a significant contribution from the lower body and core. Chapter 7 outlines plyometric exercises that target the muscles of the core. However, the summation of forces produced from the ground up in many of these movements is ultimately delivered through

147

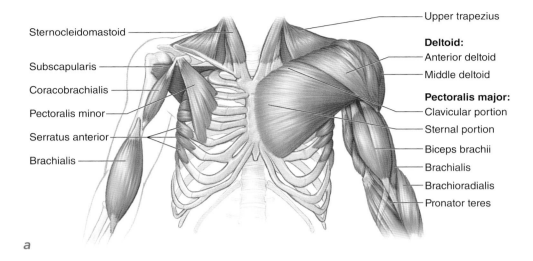

Upper trapezius

Sternocleidomastoid

Deltoid:
Anterior deltoid
Middle deltoid

Subscapularis

Coracobrachialis

Pectoralis major:
Clavicular portion
Sternal portion

Pectoralis minor

Serratus anterior

Biceps brachii

Brachialis

Brachialis

Brachioradialis

Pronator teres

a

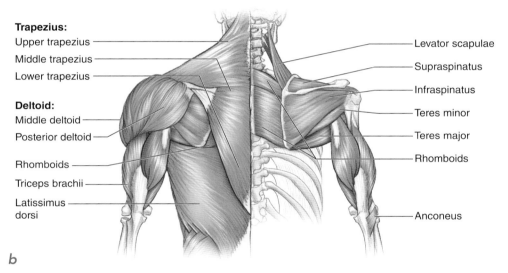

Trapezius:
Upper trapezius
Middle trapezius
Lower trapezius

Levator scapulae

Supraspinatus

Infraspinatus

Teres minor

Deltoid:
Middle deltoid
Posterior deltoid

Teres major

Rhomboids

Triceps brachii

Rhomboids

Latissimus
dorsi

Anconeus

b

FIGURE 6.1 Upper torso: *(a)* anterior; *(b)* posterior.

the upper extremities. The timing and efficient transfer of force throughout the body are imperative and necessitate close monitoring of all the muscle and joint interactions during training sessions.

The positive effects of an upper-body plyometric program cover a range of sports and specific movement patterns. The key sporting qualities improved by upper-body plyometrics training are throwing, hitting or striking a ball or opponent, propelling through water, and grappling and tackling.

Sports that involve throwing a ball or other implement require the forceful and efficient summation of forces developed from the lower body through the core and out via the upper extremities. Plyometric exercises using medicine balls or other weighed objects enhance performance for all throwing sports, whether the sport involves throwing a relatively light object (baseball, softball, American football) or throwing a heavier object (shot put, javelin, discus). Throwing a medicine ball provides a specific sequence of movements very similar to that required in all of these sports but also provides safe additional loading for the development of strength and power adaptations.

While some sports involve throwing a ball, others involve hitting a ball with either the hand (volleyball) or a piece of equipment (racket, golf club, baseball bat). In a manner similar to throwing, the arms and hands ultimately deliver the impact, but significant contributions from the lower body are important for the performance. Coordinating lower-body propulsion with a powerful transfer of force through the core and torso helps ensure the success of an explosive delivery via the hands. Performing plyometric movements with a medicine ball or similar implement reinforces the sequence of muscular contractions under heavier loads to enhance performance for sport-specific movements.

In contact or combat sports, the ability to deliver a powerful punch or strike with the hands is extremely important. Explosive movements that involve a dynamic pushing motion improve striking abilities, particularly when combined with a powerful contribution from the lower body. Medicine-ball push throws or reactive push-ups are commonly used to improve upper-body striking.

Swimmers rely on the arms for a large portion of their propulsion abilities in the water. Generating large amounts of force through the water requires significant strength and power and the durability to last through long workout sessions on consecutive training days. While specific muscular endurance capabilities are important for success in swimming and related activities, upper-body power is critical for maintaining optimal technique in the water.

Combat sports such as wrestling, judo, and mixed martial arts require significant strength and power for grappling with opponents for long training sessions and intense matches. Rugby and football players need the same arm strength for tackling opponents consistently under high-speed conditions. Explosive activities that involve pulling movements enhance both grappling and tackling performance by improving overall efficiency in muscle recruitment and general strength.

DYNAMIC PUSH-UP EXERCISES

Push-ups are a traditional body-weight exercise for developing overall strength and power for pushing movements, targeting the muscles of the chest (pectoralis major), shoulders (anterior deltoid), and arms (triceps brachii). The addition of rapid acceleration and deceleration through dynamic movements can significantly increase the load on these muscles as well as prepare them for the explosive demands of sport. Dynamic push-up exercises can build concentric abilities for pushing movements, eccentric strength qualities for resisting movement, and plyometric qualities for reactive abilities. Because dynamic push-up exercises can place a great deal of stress on the shoulder joints, you should follow a gradual progression of work to minimize the risk of injury.

MEDICINE-BALL PASSES AND THROWS

Use medicine balls to develop upper-body strength, power, and elasticity through a variety of passes and throws. Throwing the medicine ball back and forth with a partner is a productive and fun activity. When a partner is not available, throw the medicine ball against a solid wall structure to develop athletic upper-body qualities. The decision to use partner throws rather than wall throws depends on availability of equipment and facilities as well as the objectives of the training session. In cases where it is desirable to have a more rapid and predictable return of the medicine ball for individual repetitions of throws, using a wall for these exercises may be more appropriate. Where interaction with another athlete creates less predictable flight paths for the incoming medicine ball—simulating actual sporting scenarios—partner throws may be more desirable.

Selecting an appropriate medicine ball for chosen activities is an important step in the process. The ball must be constructed of a material that is easy to grip and also provides some degree of cushioning, or give. A ball that is too hard is not only harder to catch but also very stressful on the hands over numerous repetitions. Conversely, a ball that is too soft may not provide enough bounce for rebounding throws against a wall. Smaller medicine balls may be difficult to catch, but larger medicine balls can be difficult to throw. Finally, the weight of the medicine ball must be appropriate for you and your chosen exercise. When in doubt, always opt for a slightly lighter ball for safety and the preservation of movement quality.

UPPER-BODY EXERCISES USING OTHER EQUIPMENT

You can use many other types of equipment to create optimal training adaptations for dynamic upper-body movements. Having a variety of training equipment cannot only create additional sport-specific training adaptations but also provide a more stimulating training environment for athletes who can easily get bored through excessive repetition. Kettlebells can be used to create dynamic swinging motions that develop power and strength in the posterior muscles of the upper body. A suspended heavy bag used by boxers can be integrated into explosive pushing movements in a manner that maximizes safety with heavier loads.

REACTIVE WALL PUSH-UP

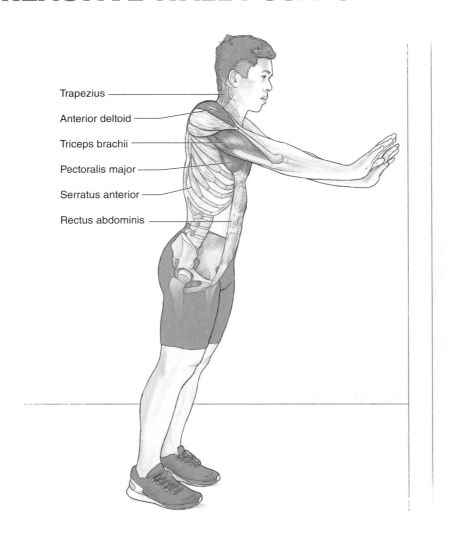

Trapezius

Anterior deltoid

Triceps brachii

Pectoralis major

Serratus anterior

Rectus abdominis

Execution

1. Stand approximately 24 to 40 inches (60 to 100 cm) away from a solid wall structure with the feet hip-width apart and directly face the wall. Bring the hands up and hold in a ready position at chest height to prepare for contact with the wall.

2. Fall forward toward the wall, maintaining a tall standing posture. Hands contact the wall with elbows at the sides of the body. Decelerate the body's forward fall for a short range of motion.

3. Reverse the direction of the body's fall with a forceful push with both hands. Extend the elbows explosively to return to a fully standing position. Repeat.

Muscles Involved

Primary: Pectoralis major, triceps brachii, anterior deltoid.

Secondary: Serratus anterior, trapezius, rectus abdominis.

Exercise Notes

Reactive wall push-ups are an effective upper-body plyometric movement for beginner and intermediate athletes who would like to develop dynamic strength safely. This exercise builds strength, power, and elastic abilities in the chest, shoulders, and triceps with lower loads than a conventional dynamic push-up performed on the floor. The overall load experienced during the wall push-up can be adjusted by the angle of body alignment. A taller posture relative to the wall will yield lower overall forces than a flatter body posture. It is advisable to start with a taller posture if you're less advanced and then progress to a lower angle once strength and power improve.

VARIATION

Reactive Push-Up With Box

To place the body at a lower angle relative to the floor, perform reactive push-ups onto a raised bench or box. Instead of falling toward the box from a standing position, start from an extended push-up position with the hands on the box. Flex the elbows and permit the downward acceleration of the body toward the top of the box. Reverse the direction of the fall with a powerful push-up. Complete as individual repetitions with a pause or as a continuous rebounding exercise.

EXPLOSIVE PUSH-UP

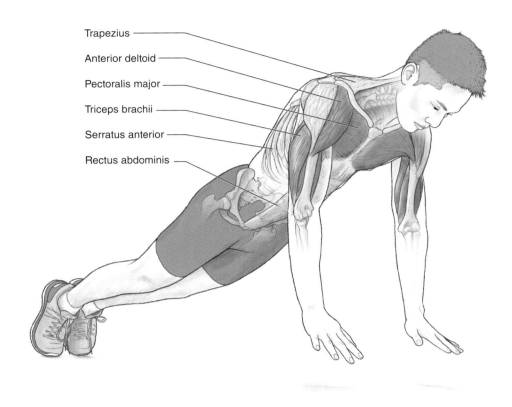

Trapezius

Anterior deltoid

Pectoralis major

Triceps brachii

Serratus anterior

Rectus abdominis

Execution

1. Begin with the body flat on the floor in the bottom of a push-up position with arms placed slightly wider than shoulder-width and feet close to each other.

2. Powerfully push the body up off the floor by applying force to the floor, extending through the full range of motion for the pushing action.

3. Once the body reaches the top of the motion and begins to descend to the floor, prepare the hands to contact the floor and decelerate the body in a controlled manner back to the floor.

Muscles Involved

Primary: Pectoralis major, triceps brachii, anterior deltoid.

Secondary: Serratus anterior, trapezius, rectus abdominis.

Exercise Notes

Explosive push-ups involve the acceleration of the body upward with a forceful pushing motion from the arms. The intent is to create enough force to fully extend the elbows rapidly and create some degree of separation of the hands from the ground. The full motion includes a powerful concentric phase and a strong eccentric landing phase to decelerate the body. Perform no more than 6 repetitions of this exercise to retain maximum force through the set. An emphasis on good technical execution is imperative for maintaining efficient mechanics and minimizing the risk of injury.

VARIATION

Explosive Push-Up to Raised Boxes

The explosive push-up to raised boxes can be considered the upper-body equivalent of a box jump. The explosive upward push launches the body onto raised platforms or low boxes. Using such equipment provides a performance goal for each repetition and reduces landing impacts at the completion of each explosive effort. Boxes should be low enough and appropriately stable to allow a safe landing. The optimal location of the boxes is on either side of the hands to allow for a smooth transition from the starting position. Start with the body flat on the floor and hands by the sides of the torso. Push explosively into the floor and land with the hands on each box. Carefully walk the hands back to the floor and reset the starting position between each repetition with the body position flat on the ground.

DROP-AND-CATCH PUSH-UP

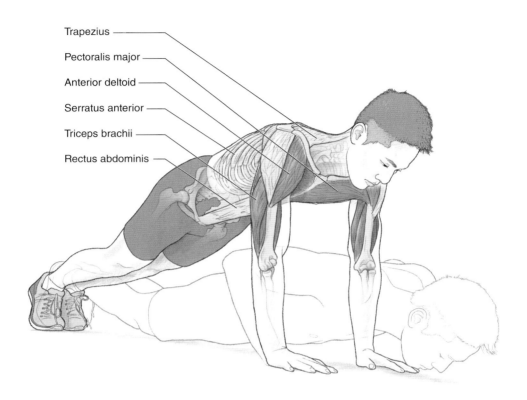

Trapezius

Pectoralis major

Anterior deltoid

Serratus anterior

Triceps brachii

Rectus abdominis

Execution

1. Begin in an extended push-up position with arms slightly wider than shoulder-width apart and feet close to each other, similar to a plank position.
2. To allow the body to drop to the floor, shuffle the hands outward rapidly and allow the elbows to flex during the downward motion.
3. Catch the body a few inches from the floor with the hands firmly planted alongside the torso. Slowly perform a push-up movement to reposition the body back up to the starting position and repeat the exercise.

Muscles Involved

Primary: Pectoralis major, triceps brachii, anterior deltoid.

Secondary: Serratus anterior, trapezius, rectus abdominis.

Exercise Notes

The drop-and-catch push-up for the upper body is similar to a drop jump from a box that targets the lower body. The intent is to harness the maximal muscle recruitment capabilities of the muscles in the upper extremities, shoulders, and chest through use of a strong eccentric contraction. Keep the number of repetitions low (3 to 6), especially if you are new to the exercise. You also can drop to various ranges of motion, depending on the specific demands of your sport. For example, an offensive lineman in American football may want to build resistive strength to a specific range of motion in front of the body so that his arms do not collapse backward when he makes contact with an opposing defensive lineman. You can customize this push-up to fit the demands of a specific player and the objectives outlined by a sport coach.

VARIATION

Drop-and-Catch Push-Up From Box

Starting a drop-and-catch push-up from a higher position generates greater eccentric forces. Place low boxes on either sides of the hands to serve as the starting position for the exercise. Quickly shift the hands inward and allow the body to accelerate to the floor. The landing will be more forceful than the standard drop-and-catch push-up. Take special care to decelerate the body safely to the floor.

REACTIVE FLOOR PUSH-UP

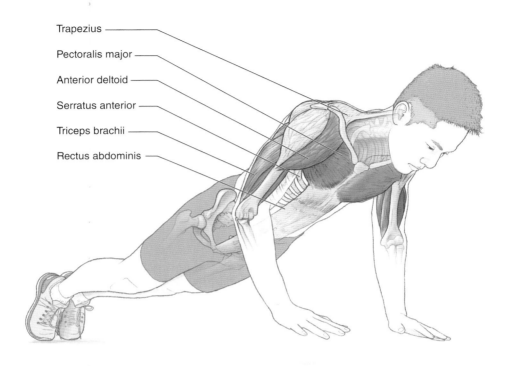

Trapezius

Pectoralis major

Anterior deltoid

Serratus anterior

Triceps brachii

Rectus abdominis

Execution

1. Start on the floor with the hands beside the body at approximately shoulder width.

2. Powerfully push into the floor to drive the body upward. As the body rises, ensure the elbows reach full extension. Depending on the amount of force delivered during the push, the hands may leave the floor but it is not necessary to become airborne.

3. Descend to the floor with the hands prepared for ground contact and a smooth deceleration phase. As muscle tension develops in the arms, shoulders, and chest, quickly reverse the direction of movement from down to up, pushing the body back to its highest position.

4. The dynamic repetitions occur in a rebounding fashion off the floor with consistent velocity and height.

Muscles Involved

Primary: Pectoralis major, triceps brachii, anterior deltoid.

Secondary: Serratus anterior, trapezius, rectus abdominis.

Exercise Notes

Reactive floor push-ups can be considered the upper-body equivalent of a repetitive squat jump. The objective is to powerfully launch the torso upward over a number of repetitions, taking advantage of the elastic properties of the shoulders, triceps, and chest muscles. You can drop to a position just above the floor or reverse the direction of movement from a higher position, depending on the range of motion desired. Because of the forceful nature of reactive floor push-ups, limit the total number of repetitions per set to 6. Monitor body posture and time spent on the floor to identify fatigue and determine the optimal volume of work.

VARIATION

Reactive Push-Up With Narrow Hand Position

Shifting the hand position inward for the reactive floor push-up requires greater contribution from the triceps. Begin by shifting to a position slightly inside shoulder width. Avoid hand spacing that is too narrow; this may place excessive stress on the elbows and affect overall stability of landings. When transitioning to a narrow hand position, use fewer repetitions until you develop greater confidence and strength.

CLAPPING PUSH-UP

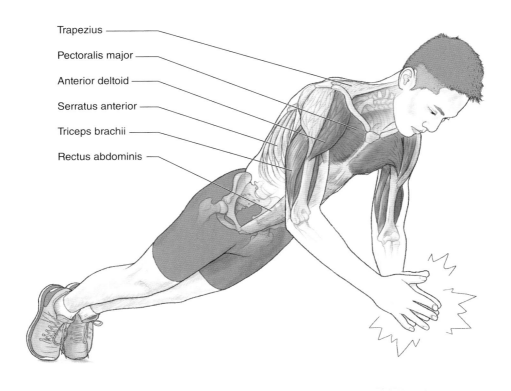

Trapezius

Pectoralis major

Anterior deltoid

Serratus anterior

Triceps brachii

Rectus abdominis

Execution

1. Begin in an extended push-up position with arms slightly wider than shoulder width and feet close to each other.

2. Lower the body quickly in a controlled manner. Reverse the direction of motion with a forceful pushing action while keeping the feet on the floor.

3. With the torso suspended in the air, clap the hands together quickly and then catch the body in a standard push-up position. Pause before repeating or perform all repetitions using a rebounding motion.

Muscles Involved

Primary: Pectoralis major, triceps brachii, anterior deltoid.

Secondary: Serratus anterior, trapezius, rectus abdominis.

Exercise Notes

Clapping push-ups are an advanced upper-body plyometric exercise that places significant loads on the shoulders, arms, and chest. A powerful pushing motion should create adequate separation from the ground to allow the hands to clap in front of the chest. The dynamic nature of this intense exercise builds general strength and elastic power in the upper extremities and chest. Use fewer repetitions—4 to 6 per set—to ensure that the quality of the movement and maximal effort is maintained.

VARIATION

Clapping Push-Up From Knees

If clapping push-ups from the feet are too difficult, modify the exercise to provide a base of support from the knees. This modification places significantly less stress on the arms and chest. You can still perform explosive clapping push-ups from your knees before progressing to the full exercise.

SINGLE-ARM PUSH PASS

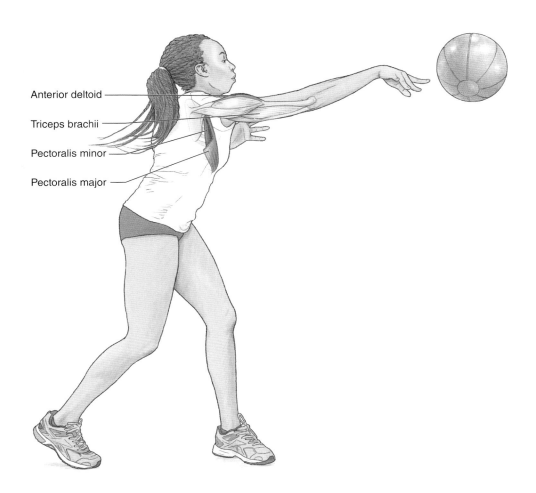

Anterior deltoid

Triceps brachii

Pectoralis minor

Pectoralis major

Execution

1. From a tall standing position with feet hip-width apart, draw the medicine ball in toward one shoulder. Choose a distance between yourself and the wall or partner that allows for a powerful push that reaches the desired target.

2. Push the ball powerfully forward with the elbow extending fully through the release of the ball.

3. If you are throwing the ball against a wall, stand close enough to the wall to ensure the ball returns to the location of the shoulder. Partner throws should be directed to a partner's shoulder.

4. Repeat the throw with the same arm or switch to the opposite arm through the set.

Muscles Involved

Primary: Pectoralis major, pectoralis minor, anterior deltoid.

Secondary: Triceps brachii.

Exercise Notes

The single-arm push pass is a concentric pushing exercise that develops basic unilateral strength and power in the upper extremities. This motion is valuable for sports such as boxing and basketball, where a quick jabbing or pushing motion is desired without a time-consuming gather motion or countermovement. Perform a quick, pulsing motion, creating as much velocity on the throw as possible. It is critical to select a ball of an appropriate weight to maintain velocity; a slightly lighter ball is recommended initially. Use higher volumes of 10 to 12 repetitions per arm for these powerful pulsing passes.

VARIATION

Rotating Single-Arm Push Pass

To provide added force behind the single-arm push pass, rotate the shoulders and gather for each individual throw. You also can use the lower body to develop force from the ground. Force travels through the core and out the shoulder. The momentum of the incoming medicine ball, delivered from either a partner throw or a wall throw rebound, loads the muscles and tendons of the chest and shoulder to create greater local force and induce torso rotation and greater contribution from the lower body for successive throws. These throws are especially useful for athletes who actively wind up before striking a ball such as in tennis and other racket-based sports.

SINGLE-LEG STANDING PUSH PASS

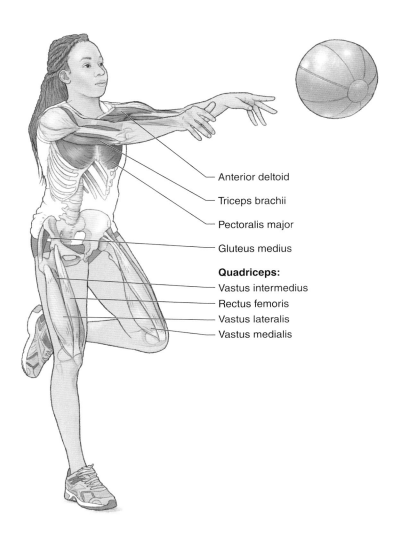

Anterior deltoid

Triceps brachii

Pectoralis major

Gluteus medius

Quadriceps:
Vastus intermedius
Rectus femoris
Vastus lateralis
Vastus medialis

Execution

1. Stand on one leg opposite a partner or a wall. Start with the medicine ball at chest height and the elbows beside the rib cage.

2. Forcefully push the medicine ball away from the body, maintaining balance in the single-leg stance. With a throw to a partner, maintain a regular rhythm of moderate- to high-velocity throws that are returned to the chest area. In the case of throws against a wall, stand close enough to the wall to ensure that powerful throws are returned at chest height.

3. As you receive the medicine ball, decelerate the ball with the hands as it approaches the body. Maintain balance and control on the supporting single leg. Complete the prescribed number of repetitions on one leg, then switch to the other leg.

Muscles Involved

Primary: Pectoralis major, anterior deltoid, triceps brachii.

Secondary: Gluteus medius, quadriceps (rectus femoris, vastus lateralis, vastus intermedius, vastus medialis).

Exercise Notes

A single-leg standing push pass works the upper body while requiring you to maintain lower-body stability and proprioception. The harder the push throw, the greater the demands on the lower body to provide a stable base. When throwing the medicine ball back and forth with a partner, target the throws to either side of the midline of the body to place greater demands on the supporting leg. Because these throws will not be as powerful as bilateral-stance throws, you can perform more repetitions (10 to 15 throws) to build specific muscular endurance in the stance leg.

VARIATION

Explosive Single-Leg Push Pass

You can perform explosive push passes from a single-leg stance, generating a significant amount of force from the lower body culminating in a powerful two-hand throw of the medicine ball. Start in a low crouch position on a single leg, holding the ball in front of the body at chest height. Begin the movement with the powerful extension of the hip, knee, and back to full extension before pushing the ball with the hands. The explosive single-leg push pass can finish with a double-leg landing.

EXPLOSIVE SQUAT THROW

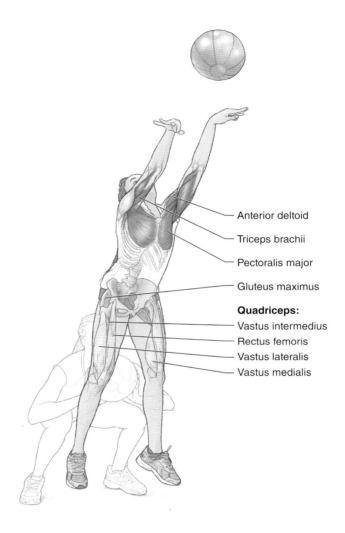

Anterior deltoid

Triceps brachii

Pectoralis major

Gluteus maximus

Quadriceps:
Vastus intermedius
Rectus femoris
Vastus lateralis
Vastus medialis

Execution

1. Begin the exercise with a tall posture. Position the feet shoulder-width apart. Hold the medicine ball in front of the body against the chest.

2. Perform a countermovement, descending to a half-squat position with the knees at 90 degrees flexion, in an effort to generate additional force from the lower body. Maintain a relatively upright posture with the torso.

3. Extend vertically from the knees and hips, accelerating the body upward similar to a squat jump. It is not uncommon for the feet to leave the ground if the throwing effort is powerful enough.

4. At the top of the squat, push the medicine ball powerfully overhead for maximum height. Allow the ball to fall to the ground, then repeat.

Muscles Involved

Primary: Pectoralis major, anterior deltoid, triceps brachii.

Secondary: Gluteus maximus, quadriceps (rectus femoris, vastus lateralis, vastus intermedius, vastus medialis).

Exercise Notes

Explosive squat throws work on vertical force production for both the upper and lower body. The movement begins with a powerful contribution from the lower body, transferring to an explosive upper-body vertical throw. This exercise is useful for developing general vertical explosive abilities and specific movements in sports. Basketball players who drive upward with a ball to the hoop will benefit from this exercise. Volleyball players working on blocking skills also can develop greater power and overall extension above the net.

VARIATION

Squat Jump Into Squat Throw

Perform one or two explosive squat jumps before performing an explosive squat throw. The combination of jumps and throws reinforces the similarity in the execution of each exercise; the jumps prepare you for a powerful squat throw. The initial squat jumps can be maximal or submaximal, depending on the total number of repetitions in a single set. The intent is to create a scenario in which the squat throw performance is maximized for each repetition.

UNDERHAND VERTICAL SQUAT THROW

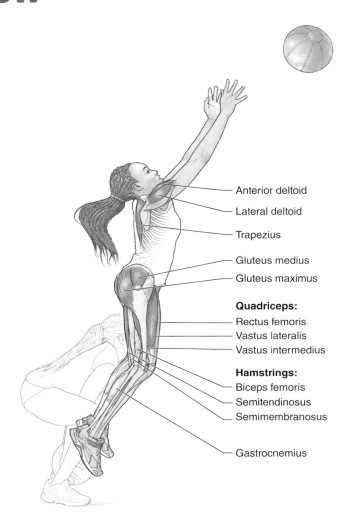

- Anterior deltoid
- Lateral deltoid
- Trapezius
- Gluteus medius
- Gluteus maximus

Quadriceps:
- Rectus femoris
- Vastus lateralis
- Vastus intermedius

Hamstrings:
- Biceps femoris
- Semitendinosus
- Semimembranosus

- Gastrocnemius

Execution

1. Stand in a tall posture. Hold the medicine ball in front of the body at waist height.
2. Descend into a low squat, keeping the torso upright, arms extended, and ball in front of the body to generate additional force from the lower body.
3. Extend vertically from the knees and hips, accelerating the body upward similar to a squat jump movement. If enough force is generated during the throw, it is common for the feet to leave the ground. Maintain an extended arm position through the jump.

4. At the top of the squat, pull the medicine ball powerfully upward along the body for maximum height on the throw. The trajectory of the throw can be vertical or slightly forward, particularly if passing to a partner.

5. The body can extend off the floor at the end of the throw, particularly if it is a powerful effort. Make sure the ball does not hit you when it falls back down.

Muscles Involved

Primary: Trapezius, lateral deltoid, anterior deltoid, gluteus maximus, gluteus medius, semitendinosus, vastus lateralis, vastus medialis, vastus intermedius.

Secondary: Gastrocnemius, biceps femoris, semimembranosus, rectus femoris.

Exercise Notes

The underhand vertical squat throw can be an explosive exercise at maximal intensity or a general strength activity performed at submaximal intensity. The maximal heave throw develops upper-body pulling power for sports such as rowing and wrestling. The lower-body contributions can be helpful for overall starting strength and vertical jumping ability. As with many throws, the combination of lower-body power at the beginning of the movement and upper-body speed toward the end of the throw produces a high-velocity performance that launches the ball for maximum distance. Launch the ball along the front of the body in a vertical path. For maximal efforts, perform 6 to 8 repetitions in each set. For submaximal throws, perform 8 to 15 repetitions in each set. When you cannot perform Olympic weightlifting movements, maximal heave throws for height are a viable substitute for developing vertical power.

VARIATION

Underhand Vertical Squat Throw With Jumps

Perform multiple squat jumps before the underhanded vertical squat throw to add intense movement. In some cases, one or two submaximal jumps before a maximal throw prepares the muscles for one exceptional effort on the throw. Hold the medicine ball directly above the head for the preparatory jumps and then drop the ball to below waist level to deliver the final throw. Perform 4 or 5 throws per set to develop vertical force.

SPLIT-STANCE SCOOP THROW

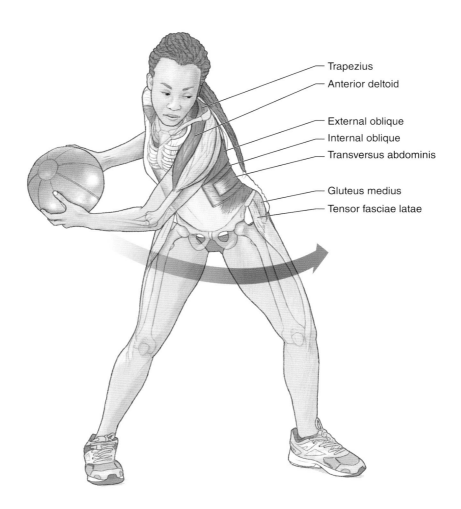

Trapezius
Anterior deltoid
External oblique
Internal oblique
Transversus abdominis
Gluteus medius
Tensor fasciae latae

Execution

1. Start in a moderate split stance with the feet approximately 12 to 16 inches (30 to 40 cm) apart from heel to toe. The stance width can be similar to the width of the shoulders. Maintain an upright posture, holding the medicine ball to one side of the body with the arms extended.

2. Draw the medicine ball back past the rear hip and then throw the ball forcefully in a powerful underhand scoop throw to a partner or against a solid wall. The partner returns the ball to the height of the midsection. If using a wall throw, stand close enough to the wall to have the ball returned to waist height with a powerful throw.

3. Repeat the throw in a rhythmic fashion on one side, then switch to the other side for the next set.

Muscles Involved

Primary: Trapezius, anterior deltoid, transversus abdominis, internal oblique, external oblique, multifidus.

Secondary: Gluteus medius, erector spinae (iliocostalis, longissimus, spinalis), tensor fasciae latae.

Exercise Notes

This underhand throw is a good exercise for enhancing rotational power from a split stance. Strength and stability in the lower body are combined with dynamic power and mobility through the core and upper body. You can do this exercise as a rhythmic set of circuit passes for general strength and fitness or as a more explosive throw to develop rotational power. Establish a good base of support in the split stance.

VARIATION

Drop Split Into Scoop Throw

Stand tall and drop into a split position, with the front thigh parallel to the ground, before the scoop throw for a more dynamic version of this exercise. The drop into a split stance loads the lower body and uses elastic strength properties before a powerful scoop throw. Make sure not to split into a stance so deep that the knee of the rear leg contacts the ground. These types of dynamic movements into throws are useful for sports that require reactive footwork in order to achieve a better position for receiving a ball such as in volleyball, tennis, squash, and badminton.

LATERAL SINGLE-ARM PUSH PASS

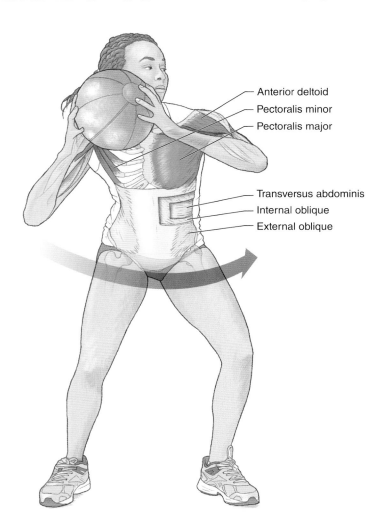

Anterior deltoid

Pectoralis minor

Pectoralis major

Transversus abdominis

Internal oblique

External oblique

Execution

1. Stand sideways to the direction of the throw with the feet shoulder-width apart, knees slightly flexed, and torso upright. Hold the medicine ball at shoulder height on one side of the body.
2. Forcefully rotate the shoulder with the medicine ball back to prestretch the muscles of the upper body and core.

3. Initiate the throw from the lower body with the feet applying force through the ground. As the movement transfers up through the body, rotate the throwing shoulder forward powerfully and extend the elbow powerfully to launch the medicine ball across the body. The partner returns the ball to the height of the shoulder. If doing a wall throw, stand close enough to the wall to have the ball returned to shoulder height with a powerful throw.

4. Multiple repetitions can begin with a catch at shoulder height, initiating the backward rotation before the throw. Establish a rhythmic pattern with partner throws or passes against a wall. Switch sides after each set.

Muscles Involved

Primary: Pectoralis major, pectoralis minor, anterior deltoid.

Secondary: Transversus abdominis, internal oblique, external oblique, multifidus, triceps brachii.

Exercise Notes

The lateral positioning of this push throw allows for strong rotational movement across the body. While the movement is similar to a punching motion, it is not a forward punch or jab. It is similar to a crossing punch. The rotation of the torso and shoulders stretches the muscles of the core and allows for greater force production. For best results, pass through the entire range of motion to best take advantage of the contribution of all anatomical structures from top to bottom. Repetitions should be fluid and quick, with a snapping motion at the end of the throw. The muscle recruitment pattern is similar to that used by an American football lineman attempting to push past a blocking opponent or a basketball player using the arms to get around a pick.

VARIATION

Lateral Push Pass From a Lunge

Lateral push passes from a lunge position place greater demands on the core and upper body. Pass across the thigh of the inside leg or the outside leg; perform sets from both positions. Set the lunge position with a stance that separates the feet by approximately 12 to 20 inches (30 to 50 cm) from heel to toe and shoulder-width apart. Throws and passes should be forceful but quick. Maintain vertical stability throughout the exercise.

KNEELING LATERAL UNDERHAND PASS

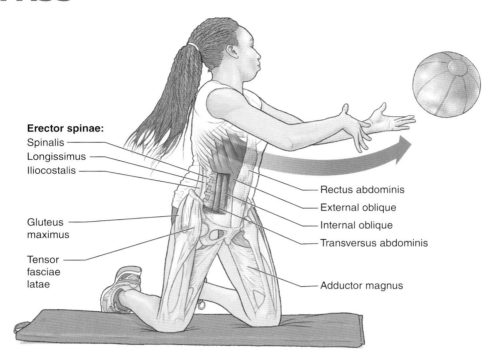

Erector spinae:
Spinalis
Longissimus
Iliocostalis

Gluteus maximus

Tensor fasciae latae

Rectus abdominis
External oblique
Internal oblique
Transversus abdominis

Adductor magnus

Execution

1. Get into a kneeling position perpendicular to the direction of the throw. Hold the medicine ball in front of the body at waist height. The throw can be to a partner or against a solid wall. Kneel on a soft surface or with an appropriate pad or exercise mat beneath the knees.

2. Draw the ball away from the direction of the throw, rotating the shoulders relative to the hips to prestretch the muscles of the core.

3. Throw the medicine ball powerfully across the body with the path of the ball close to the abdomen. Follow through with the arms and shoulders on the release of the ball.

4. When receiving the ball from a partner or a rebound off the wall, catch the ball in advance of the body and rotate back to the far side of the body to prepare for the next throw.

5. Perform on one side of the body in one set, then switch to the other side for the next set.

Muscles Involved

Primary: Transversus abdominis, internal oblique, external oblique, multifidus.

Secondary: Rectus abdominis, erector spinae (iliocostalis, longissimus, spinalis), tensor fasciae latae, adductor magnus, gluteus maximus.

Exercise Notes

A lateral pass from the knees requires greater rotation and mobility through the core to achieve appropriate range of motion in both the gather and delivery phases than a standing lateral pass. The pull of the medicine ball across the body should be powerful, making use of the force-generating abilities of both the upper body and core. Perform quick passes close to a wall or partner or pass in a forceful manner with greater distance required on each throw.

VARIATION

Kneeling Rotational Pass Behind

An even greater range of motion is required to turn the shoulders to enable a rotating pass behind the body from the kneeling position. A partner stands behind you, slightly off to one side to receive the pass. The return pass from the partner provides additional momentum for the countermovement to the opposite side of the body, generating greater force for individual passes. The rotational passes need not be maximal because the main intent is to achieve greater range of motion through repetitive throws in a strong, rhythmic fashion.

KNEELING MEDICINE-BALL OVERHEAD PASS

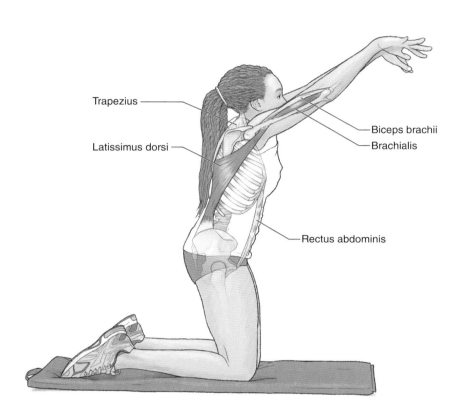

Trapezius

Latissimus dorsi

Biceps brachii

Brachialis

Rectus abdominis

Execution

1. Begin the exercise from a bilateral kneeling position on a soft surface.

2. Draw the medicine ball behind the head and then pass powerfully to a partner or against a firm wall.

3. Use a lighter medicine ball and a closer distance between yourself and your partner or the wall for easier passes from the kneeling position because throwing from this position places greater stress on the arms and shoulders.

4. Receive the ball from a partner throw or wall rebound at the point of initial release. Once the catch is made above the head, allow the ball to draw back behind the head to load the primary muscles to stretch in preparation for the next throw.

5. Maintain a firm posture throughout the exercise with a strong, stable stance from the kneeling position.

Muscles Involved

Primary: Latissimus dorsi, brachialis.

Secondary: Rectus abdominis, trapezius, biceps brachii.

Exercise Notes

A kneeling medicine-ball overhead pass places a greater load on the upper body and core than a standing pass. Shorter passes with lower throw velocities are to be expected from the kneeling position than from the standing position, where more muscles and joints are involved in the summation of force for the throwing action.

VARIATION

Falling Kneeling Medicine-Ball Overhead Pass

Falling forward as part of the throwing motion from the knees adds force and velocity to the medicine-ball throw. Practice under submaximal conditions to ensure you can complete the throw and safely slow your fall to the ground by using your arms.

LATERAL ROTATING OVERHEAD PASS

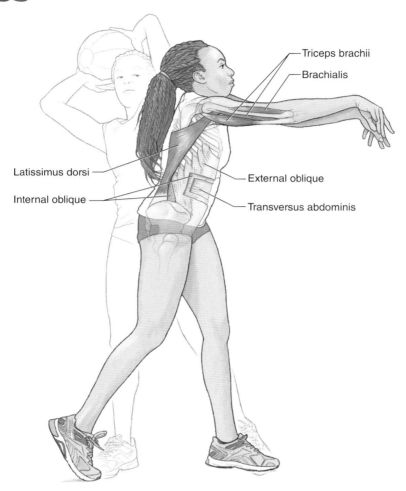

Triceps brachii

Brachialis

Latissimus dorsi

Internal oblique

External oblique

Transversus abdominis

Execution

1. Stand sideways to the direction of the throw with the feet shoulder-width apart. Hold the medicine ball directly overhead.

2. Draw the medicine ball to a position behind the head, flexing at the elbows and stretching the triceps muscles.

3. Initiate the throw by rotating the torso to one side and pulling the ball over the head and forward.

4. On delivery of the throw, the torso can bend forward to provide additional force behind the throw.

5. Work one side for a set, then switch to the opposite side for the next set.

Muscles Involved

Primary: Latissimus dorsi, brachialis, triceps brachii.

Secondary: Transversus abdominis, internal oblique, external oblique, multifidus.

Exercise Notes

The lateral rotating overhead pass combines the rotational power of the core muscles with the upper-body strength of the shoulders and arms. The turning motion and delivery are similar to that used by a baseball pitcher loading up for the delivery of a high-velocity throw. In both cases, rotational power and the use of stored elastic energy contribute to the performance of the throw.

VARIATION

Lateral Rotating Overhead Pass From Kneeling Position

Performing the same overhead pass from a kneeling position places even more emphasis on the contribution of core and upper-body muscles for a strong throw. You can bend at the waist before delivery of the throw to contribute greater force to the throw. Make sure to choose an appropriate weight for the medicine ball because throws from kneeling and seated positions place additional stresses on the shoulders. Also, choose a soft floor or field surface to avoid irritating the knees. In some cases, you might need exercise mats to provide a comfortable kneeling surface.

LATERAL OVERHEAD BASEBALL PASS

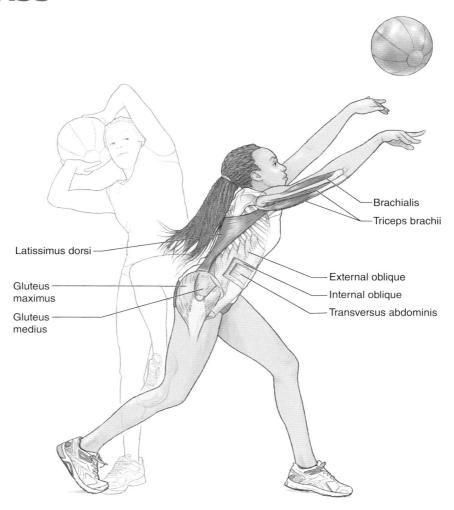

Brachialis

Triceps brachii

Latissimus dorsi

External oblique

Internal oblique

Gluteus maximus

Transversus abdominis

Gluteus medius

Execution

1. Stand sideways to the direction of the throw with the feet shoulder-width apart. Hold the medicine ball close to the body at chest height.

2. Draw the medicine ball to a position outside the shoulder farthest away from the direction of the throw. At the same time, lift the knee of the leg closest to the intended target (either a partner or a wall) to prepare for a dynamic lunge. Continue to rotate the medicine ball behind the head.

3. As the ball approaches a position behind the head, fall in the direction of the intended throw and begin to pull the ball forward over the head.

4. Deliver the throw by stepping forward with the lunging leg and powerfully pulling the ball forward with both hands.

5. Finish the throw by following through with the arms and landing in a lunge. It is common to work both sides equally with this throw to develop an overall balance in strength and mobility. You can perform this with alternating repetitions or work one side per set of throws.

Muscles Involved

Primary: Latissimus dorsi, brachialis, triceps brachii.

Secondary: Transversus abdominis, internal oblique, external oblique, multifidus, gluteus maximus, gluteus medius.

Exercise Notes

You can accomplish a more dynamic lateral overhead throw by simulating the mechanics of a throw by a baseball pitcher. Drawing the ball overhead in a semicircular motion and dropping into a lunge position on the delivery of the throw take greater advantage of elastic properties of the upper body and the momentum of the body. The timing of the mechanical components of this throw make it a much more complex movement to be used by advanced athletes. You can perform throws on one side of the body per set or in an alternating fashion within a set.

VARIATION

Overhead Baseball Pass From Lunge

As a preliminary exercise, you can perform a baseball pass from a lunging position, with one foot in front of the body and the other knee providing support on the ground. This stationary lunge position provides only the finishing position of the full lateral overhead baseball pass but allows you to focus on the upper-body portion of the throw. Less force will be produced on the throw from the lunge, and the main contribution of the throw will come from the upper extremities.

DOWNWARD SLAM THROW

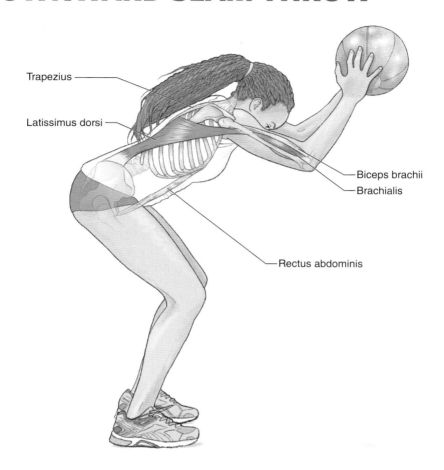

Trapezius

Latissimus dorsi

Biceps brachii

Brachialis

Rectus abdominis

Execution

1. Stand tall with feet hip-width apart. Hold the medicine ball directly overhead with the arms fully extended.
2. Initiate the movement by bending forward at the waist and dropping the torso powerfully to develop tension in the arms and shoulders.
3. Drive the ball down to the floor with the arms extended. Target a spot on the floor that is at least 12 inches away from the feet to ensure the ball does not bounce back up into your face.
4. Repeat the downward throws methodically, not rushing from repetition to repetition.

Muscles Involved

Primary: Latissimus dorsi, brachialis.

Secondary: Rectus abdominis, iliopsoas, trapezius, biceps brachii.

Exercise Notes

The downward slam throw with a medicine ball is a dynamic exercise that targets anterior musculature required for powerful swimming strokes and other sporting activities that involve throwing or grappling. The motion begins with the core musculature and is delivered by the arms. Because the throwing motion can be very stressful for the shoulders, select an appropriate medicine ball weight so you are not overloaded. Additionally, shorter repetition ranges are advisable for initial sessions to ensure technique is optimized before higher volumes of work are incorporated.

VARIATION

Rotational Downward Slam Throw

You can perform a rotational version of this exercise so that you slam the medicine ball down to either side of the body. The exercise is set up similar to a standard downward slam throw, but you begin to turn to one side once you initiate the downward motion. This variation places a greater emphasis on the oblique muscles of the core.

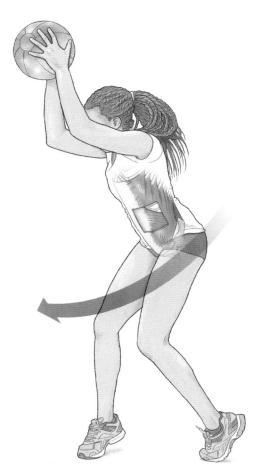

KETTLEBELL SWING

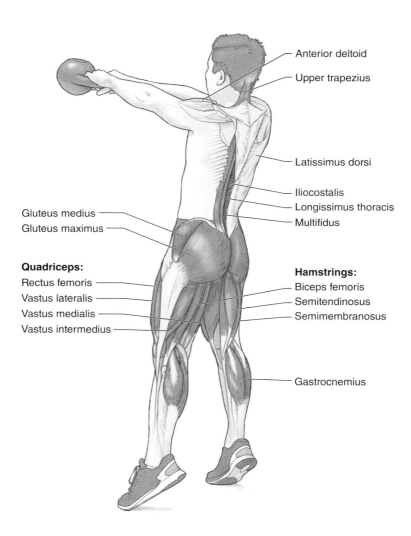

Anterior deltoid

Upper trapezius

Latissimus dorsi

Iliocostalis

Longissimus thoracis

Multifidus

Gluteus medius

Gluteus maximus

Quadriceps:
Rectus femoris
Vastus lateralis
Vastus medialis
Vastus intermedius

Hamstrings:
Biceps femoris
Semitendinosus
Semimembranosus

Gastrocnemius

Execution

1. Stand upright. Hold a kettlebell in both hands in front of the body at waist height. Place the feet in a wide stance outside the width of the shoulders with the toes pointing out slightly.

2. In the squat phase, keep the back straight and the head and eyes facing forward. During the descent, push the hips back with the kettlebell moving down and approaching the floor.

3. To initiate the swing phase, extend the kettlebell between the legs until the forearms contact the groin. Extend the hips forward and up while straightening the back to an upright position, allowing the kettlebell to move forward and upward in an arc.

4. Extend the arms upward to a point just above chest height, continuing the momentum created from the lower body and back but not straining for more height with the arms alone.

5. At the apex of the kettlebell arc, allow the weight to descend through its original arc path. Squat to accommodate the velocity and weight of the kettlebell, decelerating the weight to the same starting position between the legs.

6. Repeat for the prescribed number of repetitions.

Muscles Involved

Primary: Gluteus maximus, gluteus medius, hamstrings (semitendinosus, biceps femoris, semimembranosus), quadriceps (rectus femoris, vastus lateralis, vastus medialis, vastus intermedius), gastrocnemius.

Secondary: Anterior deltoid, multifidus, longissimus thoracis, iliocostalis, latissimus dorsi, upper trapezius.

Exercise Notes

The kettlebell swing is a good exercise for introducing a powerful pulling motion that involves the thrusting of the hips and triple extension through the ankles, knees, and hips. The transition of force production from lower body to upper body through the kettlebell swing reinforces the contribution of both regions of the body in the development of whole-body power. The dynamic movement pattern developed through the swinging of the kettlebell provides benefits for explosive running and jumping activities required in most sports.

VARIATION

Single-Arm Kettlebell Swing

Single-arm swings with a kettlebell distribute the load to an individual arm, and the body makes slight adjustments to counterbalance the asymmetrical load. The mechanics of a single-arm swing are similar to that for a double-arm swing, with the exception of some slight torso rotation at the bottom of the movement. Select an appropriate weight of kettlebell to minimize the probability of poor biomechanical execution.

HEAVY BAG PUSH

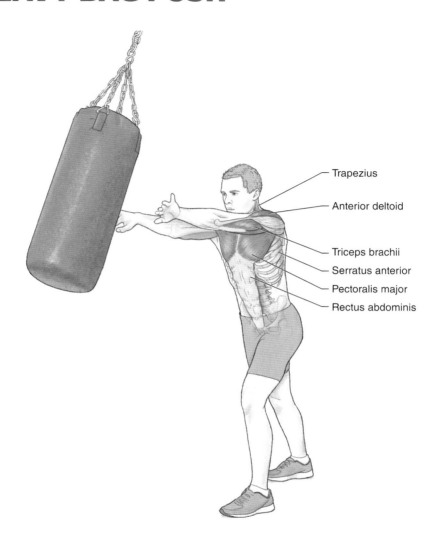

Trapezius

Anterior deltoid

Triceps brachii

Serratus anterior

Pectoralis major

Rectus abdominis

Execution

1. Stand in front of a suspended heavy punching bag with a split stance to provide greater stability during the exercise. The feet can be separated 4 to 8 inches (10 to 20 cm) from heel to toe and shoulder width.

2. Place both hands on the heavy bag with the elbows along each side of the torso. Push the heavy bag forcefully forward with maximal effort, fully extending the elbows.

3. Allow the heavy bag to swing away and back. Prepare to contact the bag with both hands. Decelerate the bag as it approaches the chest, keeping both hands on the bag with equal pressure.

4. Forcefully reverse the direction of the incoming bag with a strong push. Repeat for the prescribed number of repetitions.

Muscles Involved

Primary: Pectoralis major, triceps brachii, anterior deltoid.

Secondary: Serratus anterior, trapezius, rectus abdominis.

Exercise Notes

Using a heavy punching bag for upper-body explosive training is an effective means of preparing for the demands of contact and combat sports. Anticipating the advancing movement of the bag and preparing the hands and upper body for forceful contact involve coordination, eccentric strength, and power. The use of the stretch response in the reception and propulsion of the bag conditions the upper body in a manner that is relatively controlled and maximizes health and safety.

VARIATION

Single-Arm Heavy Bag Push

A single-arm heavy bag push trains the rotational power required for throwing or punching movements. The exercise combines lower-body strength and upper-body power to develop explosive abilities with a single arm. Continuous pushes of the heavy bag train both elastic power and overall strength qualities. Sets of single-arm heavy bag pushes should include no more than 6 repetitions per arm for explosive training. Stand beside the heavy bag with the legs set in a split position.

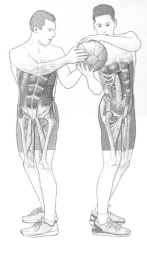

mnml# CORE
EXERCISES

N o exercise program would be complete without addressing the specific contributions of the muscles of the core and back. While the goal of any exercise program is to target specific muscles with individual movements, it can be argued that all plyometric movements rely heavily on not only the force production and transfer abilities of the core but also the ability to maintain strong posture during execution of an exercise. Thus, the abdominals (figure 7.1) and back often play a dual role: one involving dynamic movement and the other requiring strong and stable static contractions. Given the integral role of these muscles in athletic performances, you must take care to select specific exercises that recruit the core and back musculature in a manner that specifically simulates sporting movements.

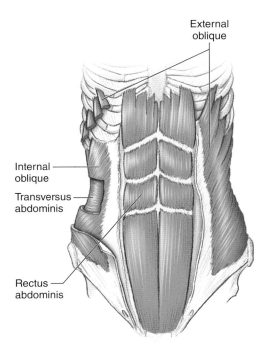

FIGURE 7.1 Abdominal muscles.

The muscles that make up the core are often classified as inner-core muscles and outer-core muscles. These classifications specify the relative location and function of the muscles. The inner-core muscles have the primary responsibility of providing stability for the midsection of the body for optimal posture and maintenance of body integrity during explosive movements. The outer-core muscles (figure 7.2) are involved in the production and assistance of dynamic movements such as sprinting, jumping, and throwing. Extension, flexion, and rotation of the torso involve the muscles of the outer core during both the production of external force and the resistance of movement through a variety of planes. Because of the complexity of sporting movements, the involvement of both inner and outer-core musculature is important at any given time and must be prepared as such.

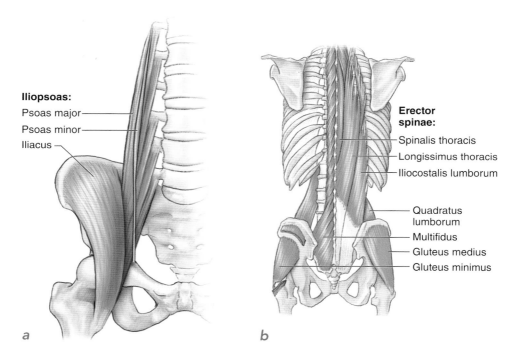

FIGURE 7.2 Outer-core muscles: *(a)* anterior; *(b)* posterior.

The inner-core muscles are composed of the transversus abdominis, multifidus, diaphragm, and pelvic floor. These muscles combine to provide support around the spine in a synergistic fashion, particularly during dynamic and explosive plyometric movements such as jumps and throws. The outer-core muscles are made up of the rectus abdominis, erector spinae group (iliocostalis, longissimus, and spinalis), and internal and external obliques. While the inner-core muscles provide stability and spinal support, the outer-core muscles assist in the production of force and power during athletic movements. All of these muscles work in a coordinated fashion whether to produce trunk flexion (rectus abdominis and iliopsoas), back extension (erector spinae combined with the hip extensors such as the glutes and hamstrings), or torso rotation and lateral flexion (internal and external obliques). All of these muscles must be trained in a balanced and coordinated fashion to not only improve athletic performance but also minimize the probability of injury.

Remember that almost every exercise identified in this book involves a significant contribution by the abdominal and back muscles, whether it involves stabilization of the spine or the production of explosive movement. The addition of specific exercises for the further development of core strength must be integrated efficiently within the overall training plan, minimizing the possibility of overuse injuries.

MEDICINE-BALL SIT-UP CHEST PASS

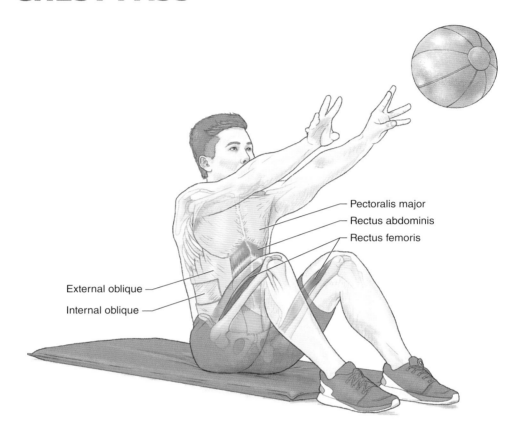

Pectoralis major
Rectus abdominis
Rectus femoris
External oblique
Internal oblique

Execution

1. Sit on the ground, holding a medicine ball at chest height in front of the body. Knees are bent at roughly 90 degrees.

2. Lower the torso to the ground in a smooth and controlled manner, keeping the medicine ball in front of the body and close to the chest.

3. Perform a strong sit-up while holding the ball in front of the body, accelerating the torso upward and forward.

4. At the top of the sit-up, powerfully push the medicine ball to a partner or against a solid wall. A partner will return the throw to the chest area for the next repetition. In the case of rebounding wall passes, the exercise should be situated close enough to the wall to allow for the return of the ball at chest height.

5. Upon return of the medicine ball, catch the ball in front of the body and bring it back toward the chest. Use the momentum of the incoming ball to drive the torso back down to the floor. Repeat a forceful sit-up motion and throw.

Muscles Involved

Primary: Rectus abdominis, iliopsoas, rectus femoris.

Secondary: Internal oblique, external oblique, pectoralis major.

Exercise Notes

The medicine-ball sit-up chest pass strengthens the outer-core muscles involved in dynamic trunk and hip flexion and requires a strong upper-body throw at the completion of the movement. This repetitive passing motion with the medicine ball can be performed with a partner or against a wall. The pushing motion at the top of the sit-up should be firm and powerful, building on the momentum of the sit-up with an explosive chest pass. When training for abdominal power, perform 6 to 8 repetitions at high velocity. For strength endurance work, perform 10 to 20 repetitions. For the initial sessions with a medicine ball, choose a 3- to 4-kilogram ball to build general strength and work capacity. As strength improves over time, you can progress to a heavier ball.

VARIATION

Overhead Medicine-Ball Sit-Up Chest Pass

Combine the sit-up motion with an overhead pass to place additional stretch on the outer-core muscles, including the rectus abdominis and psoas. Catch the medicine ball above the head, letting the momentum of the ball carry you to the ground. The ball remains extended over the head through the first half of the sit-up. The passing motion occurs at the beginning of the upward action of the sit-up with the torso following the throw. Perform repetitive throws to develop power or strength endurance. Use a relatively lighter medicine ball for the initial sessions to gradually condition the additional stretch and load created by the overhead sit-up pass.

SUPINE MEDICINE-BALL CORE PASS

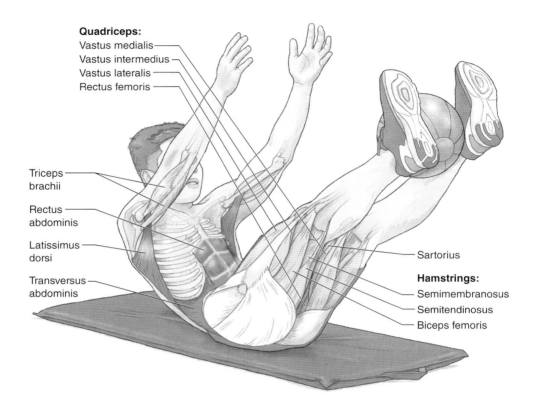

Quadriceps:
Vastus medialis
Vastus intermedius
Vastus lateralis
Rectus femoris

Triceps brachii

Rectus abdominis

Latissimus dorsi

Transversus abdominis

Sartorius

Hamstrings:
Semimembranosus
Semitendinosus
Biceps femoris

Execution

1. Lie supine with the legs outstretched and parallel to each other and the arms extended overhead holding a medicine ball.

2. Sit up, keeping the arms straight overhead, and pass the medicine ball from the hands to a position between the feet.

3. Return to the fully extended supine position with the medicine ball secured between the feet.

4. Lift the legs and ball as you sit up. Pass the ball from the feet to the hands and slowly return to the supine starting position.

5. Perform the prescribed number of repetitions in a rhythmic and controlled fashion.

Muscles Involved

Primary: Rectus abdominis, transversus abdominis, iliopsoas, latissimus dorsi.

Secondary: Sartorius, quadriceps (rectus femoris, vastus lateralis, vastus medialis, vastus intermedius), triceps brachii, hamstrings (biceps femoris, semitendinosus, semimembranosus).

Exercise Notes

The supine medicine-ball core pass is a great strength exercise for developing the core musculature but also requires a significant amount of coordination. The amount of body control and stability required for passing the weighted ball from the hands to the feet and then back again is significant and also involves flexibility through the back and hamstrings. While this exercise is not considered a dynamic core exercise, it does help develop greater overall core strength and mobility.

VARIATION

Supine Medicine-Ball Twisting Core Pass

Modify this exercise by adding a simple rotation to either side when the ball is passed from the feet to the hands. Rather than bring the ball overhead, extend the arms out to one side to stretch and recruit the internal and external oblique muscles of the core. Then draw the ball back toward the center of the body for a return pass to the feet.

MEDICINE-BALL PARTNER CRUNCH EXCHANGE

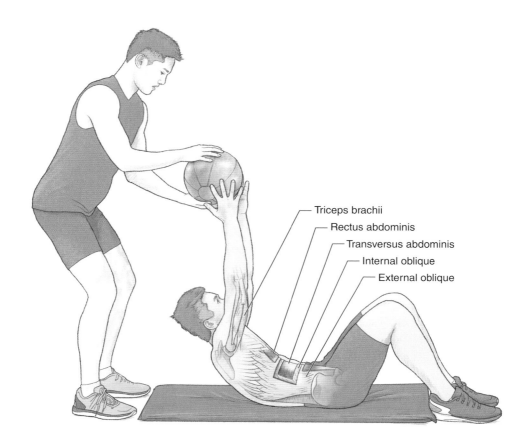

Triceps brachii
Rectus abdominis
Transversus abdominis
Internal oblique
External oblique

Execution

1. Lie supine with the legs bent at 90 degrees. A partner stands with his feet just behind your head, holding the medicine ball.

2. The partner holds the medicine ball at a height so that you have to reach up and raise your torso off the floor in order to grab the ball.

3. Reach up and grab the ball then return to the ground with the ball, keeping the arms extended.

4. On the next repetition, reach up and place the ball back into your partner's hands, then return to the ground.

5. Perform the prescribed number of repetitions in a rhythmic and controlled fashion, alternating between grabbing the ball and returning the ball.

Muscles Involved

Primary: Rectus abdominis, transversus abdominis, iliopsoas.

Secondary: Internal oblique, external oblique, triceps brachii.

Exercise Notes

The medicine-ball partner crunch exchange is a repetitive trunk-flexion exercise that involves alternating between grabbing the medicine ball and putting it back in your partner's hands on each repetition. The exercise builds general abdominal strength and can be performed over numerous repetitions to build strength endurance in the anterior muscles of the core. You can perform anywhere from 10 to 50 repetitions per set. For the initial sessions with a medicine ball, choose a 2- to 3-kilogram ball to build general strength and work capacity. As strength improves over time, progress to using a heavier ball.

VARIATION

Medicine-Ball Partner Crunch With a Moving Target

Instead of providing a consistent location for obtaining and returning the medicine ball, the partner can move the ball around. This forces you to react to the ball movement and also targets other core muscles to allow for lateral movement and some variable rotation. You may have to grab the medicine ball from above and outside the right side of your shoulder and then return it to the outside of your left shoulder. These types of variable patterns simulate actual trunk movements required in sports such as boxing.

SEATED MEDICINE-BALL LATERAL PASS

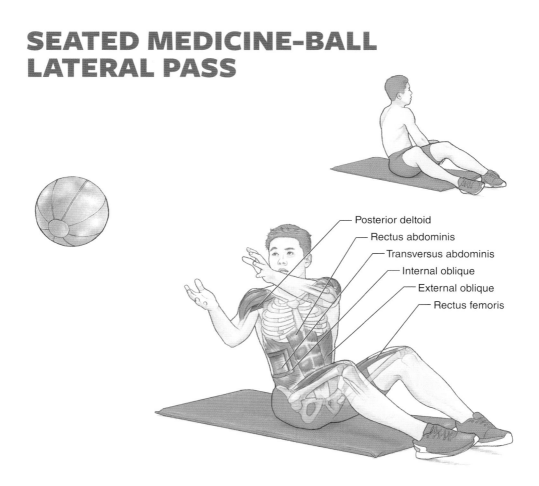

Posterior deltoid
Rectus abdominis
Transversus abdominis
Internal oblique
External oblique
Rectus femoris

Execution

1. Sit on the ground. Hold the medicine ball in front of the abdomen. Bend the knees to roughly 90 degrees.

2. Draw the ball to the opposite side of the intended direction of the pass to create a rotational countermovement with the shoulders.

3. Initiate the pass by rotating the shoulders in the direction of the pass and pulling the ball forcefully across the body to a partner or against a solid wall. A partner will return the throw to the waist area for the next repetition. In the case of rebounding wall passes, position yourself close enough to the wall to allow for the return of the ball at waist height.

4. On reception of the returning ball, allow the weight of the medicine ball to rotate the shoulders away from the direction of the pass and begin the passing sequence again.

Muscles Involved

Primary: Rectus abdominis, transversus abdominis, internal oblique, external oblique.

Secondary: Iliopsoas, posterior deltoid, rectus femoris.

Exercise Notes

Seated medicine-ball lateral passes load the core muscles with a rotational movement pattern. Your body must perform some degree of stabilization to hold the seated posture while also allowing movement through the core for the lateral pass. In this way, the exercise targets both inner- and outer-core muscles. Perform short, quick rotational passes to simulate rapid rotational movements required for sprinting or make broader, sweeping rotational passes to simulate rotational movements required for throwing sports.

VARIATION

Seated Lateral Pass With Feet Up

Simply lifting your feet off the ground for the duration of the exercise adds significant difficulty to the seated medicine-ball lateral pass. Elevating the feet off the ground more directly engages the iliopsoas and rectus femoris, placing greater responsibility for rotational movement on the rectus abdominis and oblique muscles.

SEATED MEDICINE-BALL
SEMICIRCLE PARTNER PASS

PLYOMETRIC CORE EXERCISES

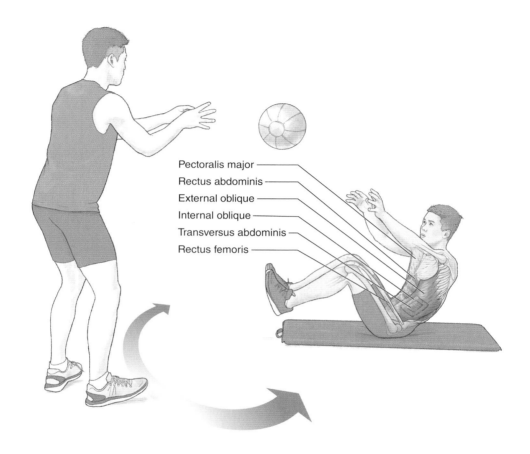

Pectoralis major
Rectus abdominis
External oblique
Internal oblique
Transversus abdominis
Rectus femoris

Execution

1. Sit on the ground. Hold the medicine ball in front of the abdomen and hold the feet a few inches above the ground.

2. Perform quick chest passes to a partner who is standing 3 to 4 feet away. Keep the feet off the ground for the duration of the exercise.

3. The partner slowly walks back and forth in a semicircle. Continue the quick passes, rotating slightly for each successive pass, adjusting to the partner's new position.

4. Perform 12 to 30 passes as your partner makes several semicircle walks back and forth.

Muscles Involved

Primary: Rectus abdominis, transversus abdominis, internal oblique, external oblique.

Secondary: Iliopsoas, rectus femoris, pectoralis major.

Exercise Notes

The seated medicine-ball semicircle partner pass builds general strength qualities in the anterior core muscles required for keeping the feet off the ground and also maintaining proper posture when passing and receiving the medicine ball. Depending on the number of repetitions used per set, general strength endurance qualities can also be developed through this exercise. You can perform anywhere from 10 to 30 passes in each set, with 3 to 5 sets in a session. The ball should be no more than 3 kilograms in the initial sessions, progressing to heavier ball weights over the course of a planned training program. The semicircle pattern traveled by a partner also forces you to rotate the torso and hold specific positions throughout the exercise.

VARIATION

Seated Rotational Partner Touches With Feet Up

In this drill, both you and your partner sit on the ground facing each other. You both keep your feet off the ground for the duration of the exercise. Start with the medicine ball. Perform 2 rotations, touching the ball to the ground for each rotation. Finish with a chest pass to your partner. Your partner performs the same number of rotating touches to the ground before passing the medicine ball back to you. You then perform 4 touches each, then 6, then 8, and then 10 touches, all while keeping your feet off the ground. Once you reach 10 repetitions, the exercise winds back down by 2 repetitions per turn until you both complete your final 2 repetitions. The pattern is 2, 4, 6, 8, 10, 8, 6, 4, 2 for both partners for one complete set. Once the pyramid repetition pattern is completed, you can rest your feet on the ground.

STANDING ROTATIONAL PARTNER PASS

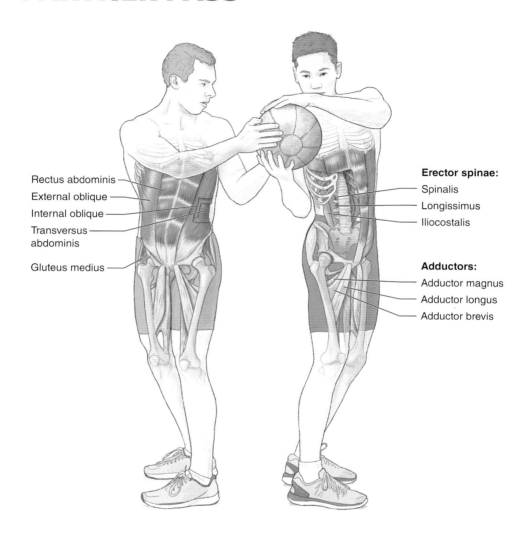

Rectus abdominis

External oblique

Internal oblique

Transversus abdominis

Gluteus medius

Erector spinae:

Spinalis

Longissimus

Iliocostalis

Adductors:

Adductor magnus

Adductor longus

Adductor brevis

Execution

1. Stand back to back with a partner approximately 1 foot apart to allow for adequate rotation of the shoulders. Hold the medicine ball at waist height in preparation for the passing movements.

2. Turn the shoulders in one direction to initiate a pass to your partner. Your partner rotates to the same side to receive the medicine ball. The exchange occurs as a hand-to-hand pass, not a throw.

3. Your partner rotates 180 degrees and passes the ball on the opposite side to complete one full revolution of the ball.

4. Continue to rotate the ball in the same direction for a prescribed number of repetitions, maintaining consistent rotational velocity and rhythm throughout the set.

5. Switch directions for the next set.

Muscles Involved

Primary: Rectus abdominis, transversus abdominis, internal oblique, external oblique.

Secondary: Gluteus medius, iliopsoas, erector spinae (iliocostalis, longissimus, spinalis), adductors (magnus, longus, brevis).

Exercise Notes

Standing rotational partner passes are a traditional core exercise that can be performed in a rhythmic fashion to develop general core strength and rotational mobility. These types of turning movements help to develop a good base of rotational coordination for agility and change of direction because the majority of these movements are initiated by trunk rotation. Passes can be performed at a steady, efficient rate without rushing the movement. Complete 10 to 15 repetitions per direction for a given set.

VARIATION

Kneeling Rotational Partner Pass

The same back-to-back exercise can be performed from a kneeling position, placing a greater emphasis for rotation on the core muscles, minimizing the contribution of the lower extremities. In both standing and kneeling variations, partners can move farther apart to modify the exercise from a short passing drill to a rotational throw, turning to the same side.

LANDMINE TRUNK ROTATION

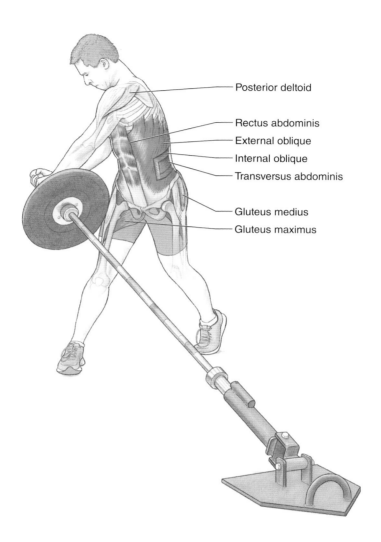

Posterior deltoid

Rectus abdominis

External oblique

Internal oblique

Transversus abdominis

Gluteus medius

Gluteus maximus

Execution

1. Load a barbell with a light to moderate weight on the upper portion. Plant the unloaded lower end of the barbell on the ground in a corner in the weight room or use a piece of equipment specifically designed for barbell landmine rotations.

2. Stand with the feet outside the width of the shoulders, with the hips and feet perpendicular to the barbell.

3. Rotate the barbell back and forth in a semicircular motion, twisting the shoulders from side to side.

4. When the barbell reaches the bottom position at approximately hip height, rebound the weight in the opposite direction, establishing an even rhythm between rotational repetitions.

Muscles Involved

Primary: Rectus abdominis, transversus abdominis, internal oblique, external oblique.

Secondary: Gluteus medius, gluteus maximus, erector spinae (iliocostalis, longissimus, spinalis), posterior deltoid.

Exercise Notes

The landmine trunk rotation is a dynamic whole-body exercise that focuses on rotational movement. A twisting motion occurs through the core between the rotating shoulder girdle and the fixed hip region of the body. The motion should be controlled but also relatively forceful to make use of the elastic strength of the core musculature. Improvement of rotational strength and power through this exercise will help in contact and combative sports when opponents must be tackled or thrown down to the ground. It can also help in throwing sports when rotational power is imperative.

VARIATION

Kneeling Landmine Trunk Rotation

To limit or remove the involvement of the lower extremities during the rotation of the barbell, kneel on a soft surface and perform the landmine exercise. The lower stance changes the barbell's semicircular path to some degree and adds some variation to the standard landmine exercise.

PRONE PUSH PASS

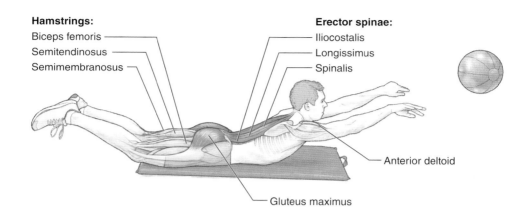

Hamstrings:
Biceps femoris
Semitendinosus
Semimembranosus

Erector spinae:
Iliocostalis
Longissimus
Spinalis

Anterior deltoid

Gluteus maximus

Execution

1. Lie prone on the ground with the ball extended in front of the head and the legs stretched out and slightly apart.
2. Simultaneously raise the torso and legs off the ground, hyperextending at the hips and back.
3. At the point of maximum hyperextension, push the medicine ball to a partner, attempting to achieve as much height and distance on the throw as possible.
4. After the release of the throw, lower the body to the start position. Have the partner gently roll the ball back and prepare for the next throw.

Muscles Involved

Primary: Erector spinae (spinalis, longissimus, iliocostalis), gluteus maximus.

Secondary: Hamstrings (biceps femoris, semitendinosus, semimembranosus), anterior deltoid.

Exercise Notes

Prone push passes are a valuable exercise for developing strength in the posterior core musculature. To counterbalance the forces created by hyperextension of the back, significant recruitment of the gluteals and hamstrings is required, resulting in the raising of the legs off the ground. The push throw of the medicine ball must be timed properly to ensure that it occurs at the highest point of torso extension, allowing for maximum height and distance on the throw. Perform no more than 8 repetitions, especially if you are new to the movement.

VARIATION

Medicine-Ball Superman Raise

If the prone pass is too difficult, you can use a less dynamic movement and still strengthen the posterior chain. Perform back extensions from the prone position while holding the medicine ball in front of the head. This serves as an introductory exercise for core and back strengthening. Perform sets of 6 to 10 repetitions to prepare for the demands of the more dynamic prone push pass. If possible, hold the hyperextension position for a few seconds to build both general strength and strength endurance.

COMBINATION PLYOMETRIC EXERCISES

While it is common for coaches and athletes to identify individual drills and exercises for achieving their performance goals and target-specific anatomy, it is also important to combine movements to better prepare athletes for the demands of their sports. Rarely does one singular jump, throw, or other explosive movement define an athletic performance, with the exception of a few track and field events and specific positions in a team sport such as a baseball pitcher. A typical athlete may run, change direction, jump, and then throw a ball in a matter of a few seconds. The speed and complexity of combined movements in a sporting scenario can occur so quickly that it is often hard to follow with the naked eye. While it is not necessary to precisely simulate these sport-specific movements, a combination of plyometric exercises can include both explosive and elastic elements found in various sports. When combined skillfully with some creativity, these exercise routines not only produce significant results but also make the training session more enjoyable.

One of the key elements of some of the combination exercises presented in this chapter is the use of sprinting. Running—in particular high-speed running—can be considered one of the purest forms of plyometric exercise. The short times of ground contact combined with high force production both horizontally and vertically found in sprinting can be of significant benefit to most, if not all, athletes. While sprinting is a useful activity for enhancing lower-body power and elasticity, when combined with other activities it can be a very effective means of improving overall performance.

Plyometric combinations fall under several categories. Jumps, throws, and sprints can be integrated to create positive adaptations for sports, enhancing overall athleticism.

MULTIPLE JUMPS

Combining a variety of jumps, whether over distance, boxes, or barriers, is an effective way of improving lower-body elastic strength, particularly when multidirectional scenarios are used. Multiple jump combinations are described and illustrated in chapter 4 using hurdles and boxes but also incorporate bilateral and unilateral jumps in the form of hopping and bounding circuits. When setting up a multijump circuit, ensure that the number of jumps is not excessive, maintaining the quality of individual foot contacts for each set. Incorporate appropriate recovery times between sets.

JUMP AND THROW

Adding one or multiple jumps before an explosive throw with a medicine ball can be useful for building lower-body power and elasticity but also reinforcing the lower-body contribution to throwing efforts. The jumps can be linear or multidirectional, ultimately finishing with a maximal throwing effort. In many respects, the jumps will build velocity, accelerate the body, and culminate in a maximal throw. The throw can be a pushing or pulling motion, depending on the emphasis of the exercise. As with all combination exercises, the integration of various movements should result in a collection of compatible efforts that easily flow into one another.

THROW AND SPRINT

The use of an explosive throw using a medicine ball before a sprint effort can enhance starting strength. While it is important to choose a medicine ball that is heavy enough to elicit a powerful throwing movement, it is also critical to ensure that the medicine ball is not so heavy that it significantly slows down the starting effort and negatively affects movement mechanics. A throw can be in the direction of the movement, such as with a push throw in the direction of a linear sprint. However, the medicine ball can also be thrown in the opposite direction of a sprint in order to work on mechanics of direction change. When combined, throws and sprints are mutually beneficial exercises that can enhance overall acceleration abilities.

An explosive throw preceding a sprint is an effective way of overloading the first movement of the running motion. Starting strength can be enhanced through the use of throw-sprint combinations. In all cases, the initial focus should be on a technically proficient and powerful throw effort with each throw followed by a high-intensity sprint. The combination of the two exercises is an effective means of improving overall starting strength and acceleration.

MULTIPLE THROWS AND SPRINTS

All types of medicine-ball throw-and-sprint combinations can be performed over longer distances using multiple throws and sprint intervals. Perform a powerful throw across a field and sprint to pick up the medicine ball and then throw it again for several sets. Powerful push throws, underhand throws, reverse overhead throws, or rotational throws may be used. In some cases, multiple types of throws can be combined, linked together by individual sprints. A push throw can start the sequence followed by a sprint. The next immediate throw could be a rotational throw on one side followed by another sprint. In many ways, it could be said that these combination drills simulate what may actually happen on a field of play, with explosive events followed by high-velocity sprints and then repeated.

In terms of developing plyometric power, multiple throws and sprints should be implemented over 6 to 10 seconds with full recovery between each set. Longer durations of combination work will begin to develop strength-endurance qualities that become less elastic and more muscular in nature.

JUMP AND SPRINT

Combining jumps and sprints as part of an exercise routine is very common and can simulate the movement requirements of many sports. Good sprinting at higher velocities will tend to have shorter ground contact times than multiple jumps. However, jumps at the start of a combination exercise can simulate the forces and ground contact times found in the early acceleration phase of sprinting, where more power is required. Thus, implementing multiple jumps that transition into the acceleration phase of running makes for a good routine when trying to improve overall power delivery on ground contact for improved sprinting abilities. Jumps can also simulate the forces found in multidirectional movements before a linear sprint effort.

Jumps preceding a sprint are a common means of either reinforcing an explosive lower-body movement as part of a starting motion or emphasizing short, elastic ground contacts. Jumps into sprints can simulate actual sport-specific movements or can emphasize qualities that contribute to faster running or more efficient movement.

Hurdles at a relatively low height can be arranged to encourage a smooth transition from bounding to sprinting. The initial series of hurdles can be higher and spread farther apart, with successive hurdles arranged lower and closer together to simulate the changes in stride length and stride frequency required for an efficient transition into a high-speed sprint.

JUMP AND THROW

When grouped into one exercise, various jump-and-throw combinations typically involve similar muscle groups. The jumping movements make use of the gluteus maximus, quadriceps, hamstrings, and calf muscles, while the throwing motions also involve the muscles of the back, deltoids, pectorals, triceps, and biceps. The summation of forces through the contribution of all of these muscle groups can create exceptional performances.

SQUAT JUMP AND MEDICINE-BALL PUSH THROW

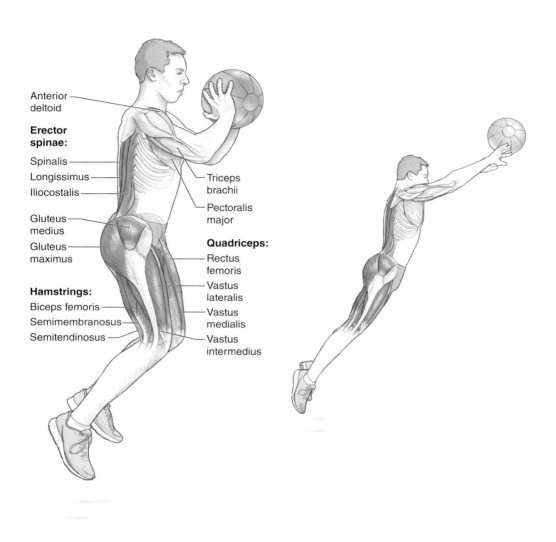

Anterior deltoid

Erector spinae:

Spinalis

Longissimus

Iliocostalis

Gluteus medius

Gluteus maximus

Hamstrings:

Biceps femoris

Semimembranosus

Semitendinosus

Triceps brachii

Pectoralis major

Quadriceps:

Rectus femoris

Vastus lateralis

Vastus medialis

Vastus intermedius

Execution

1. Stand with feet approximately shoulder-width apart. Hold the medicine ball at chest height with both hands in preparation for an explosive push throw.

2. Perform a countermovement to load the legs to prepare for a powerful jump. Initiate the jump with the intent of achieving a balance between height and distance for the flight of the jump, with a relatively upright posture.

3. Land with both feet striking the ground simultaneously midfoot. Prepare to project the body forward for the medicine-ball push throw.

4. With the medicine ball at chest height close to the body, execute a maximal throw beginning with a powerful push from the legs.

5. Finish with a high-velocity push from the arms to ensure the medicine ball achieves maximum distance.

Muscles Involved

Primary: Gluteus maximus, gluteus medius, quadriceps (rectus femoris, vastus lateralis, vastus intermedius, vastus medialis), hamstrings (biceps femoris, semitendinosus, semimembranosus), erector spinae (spinalis, longissimus, iliocostalis).

Secondary: Pectoralis major, triceps brachii, anterior deltoid.

Exercise Notes

A squat jump preceding a medicine-ball throw is a good exercise for developing lower-body power, particularly when preparing for an explosive upper-body movement such as a throw. The jump should have a good balance of distance and height to ensure the throw is supported by whole-body acceleration and activation of the stretch-shortening cycle in the lower body. The ground reaction on the landing preceding the throw will be relatively quick, converting the horizontal momentum from the jump into the push throw.

VARIATION

Multiple Squat Jumps Into a Medicine-Ball Push Throw

Combinations of two to four squat jumps can be performed over distance before an explosive medicine-ball push throw. The goal is to achieve acceleration over the series of multiple jumps, making use of lower-body power and elasticity, in an attempt to achieve a forceful throw. Over multiple jumps, keep the ball at chest height with a relatively upright posture, setting up an optimal ready position for the push throw.

SINGLE-LEG HOP AND MEDICINE-BALL PUSH THROW

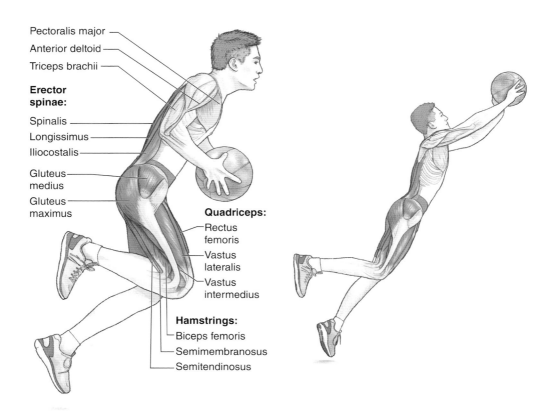

Pectoralis major
Anterior deltoid
Triceps brachii

Erector spinae:

Spinalis
Longissimus
Iliocostalis

Gluteus medius
Gluteus maximus

Quadriceps:
Rectus femoris
Vastus lateralis
Vastus intermedius

Hamstrings:
Biceps femoris
Semimembranosus
Semitendinosus

Execution

1. Stand on one leg. Hold the medicine ball at chest height with both hands in preparation for an explosive push throw.

2. Initiate a single-leg hop of moderate distance to ensure that you achieve adequate stability and control before an explosive throw.

3. Land midfoot on one leg. Maintain a relatively upright posture into the landing.

4. Perform the medicine-ball push throw from a more upright position than a bilateral push due to the lower force production from a single leg.

5. Complete the throw with a forceful push from the arms, striving for maximum distance on the effort. After completing the throw, land on both feet to maximize stability at the conclusion of the repetition.

6. Perform all repetitions on one leg and then switch legs or alternate legs with each throw.

Muscles Involved

Primary: Gluteus maximus, gluteus medius, quadriceps (rectus femoris, vastus lateralis, vastus intermedius, vastus medialis), hamstrings (biceps femoris, semitendinosus, semimembranosus), erector spinae (spinalis, longissimus, iliocostalis).

Secondary: Pectoralis major, triceps brachii, anterior deltoid.

Exercise Notes

A single-leg hop into a medicine-ball push throw focuses on developing single-leg power and elasticity. Because only one leg delivers lower-body power, the angle of the body will be more upright on delivery of the throw. After the dynamic single-leg throw, a landing on two legs is recommended.

VARIATION

Multiple Single-Leg Hops Into Medicine-Ball Push Throw

Performing a series of single-leg hops before a medicine-ball push throw allows for the accumulation of greater velocity before an explosive throw. You can apply two to five single-leg hops before a throw. Using single-leg hops will strengthen individual legs but also enhance stability in each leg in preparation for dynamic movements.

HURDLE HOPS AND MEDICINE-BALL PUSH THROW

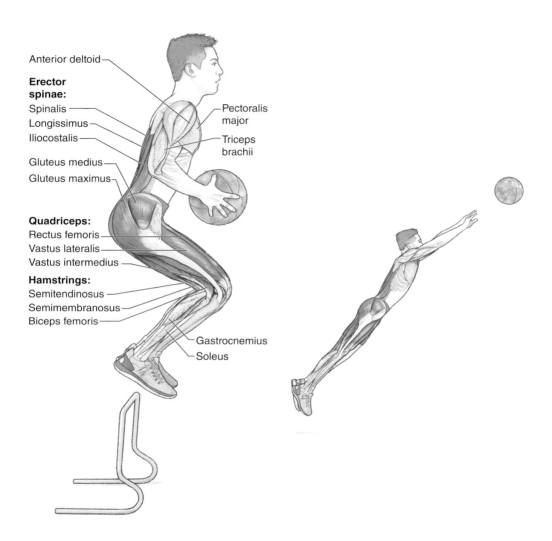

Anterior deltoid

Erector spinae:
Spinalis
Longissimus
Iliocostalis

Gluteus medius
Gluteus maximus

Quadriceps:
Rectus femoris
Vastus lateralis
Vastus intermedius

Hamstrings:
Semitendinosus
Semimembranosus
Biceps femoris

Pectoralis major

Triceps brachii

Gastrocnemius
Soleus

Execution

1. Arrange one to five hurdles in a row with adequate space between each hurdle to allow for two-foot hops.

2. Hold the medicine ball at chest height close to the body. Hop through the hurdles.

3. Ensure that the ground contacts between the hurdles are short in duration and elastic in nature.

4. After landing over the last hurdle, gather for the throw with slightly deeper knee flexion than on the previous jumps to produce a more forceful throw.

5. Complete the throw with a forceful push from the arms, striving for maximum distance on the effort.

Muscles Involved

Primary: Gluteus maximus, gluteus medius, quadriceps (rectus femoris, vastus lateralis, vastus intermedius, vastus medialis), hamstrings (biceps femoris, semitendinosus, semimembranosus), erector spinae (spinalis, longissimus, iliocostalis).

Secondary: Pectoralis major, triceps brachii, anterior deltoid, soleus, gastrocnemius.

Exercise Notes

Performing quick, elastic jumps over hurdles before an explosive medicine-ball throw will ensure jumps of uniform height and distance as part of this exercise. For initial sessions, the hurdles can be relatively low at 6 to 8 inches (15 to 20 cm). The lower hurdles will ensure quicker ground contacts and greater horizontal acceleration over the hurdles before the throw. Hurdles of greater height (18 to 30 inches, or 45 to 75 cm) can elicit more powerful jumps in succession in advance of an explosive medicine-ball throw.

VARIATION

Multidirectional Hurdle Hops Into Medicine-Ball Push Throw

You can perform a combination of linear and lateral hurdle hops in advance of an explosive medicine-ball push throw. The multidirectional hurdle hops can simulate the forces encountered during high-intensity direction changes, culminating in a powerful throwing motion. You can use lower hurdles for initial sessions with higher hurdle progressions integrated over time.

SQUAT JUMP AND REVERSE OVERHEAD MEDICINE-BALL THROW

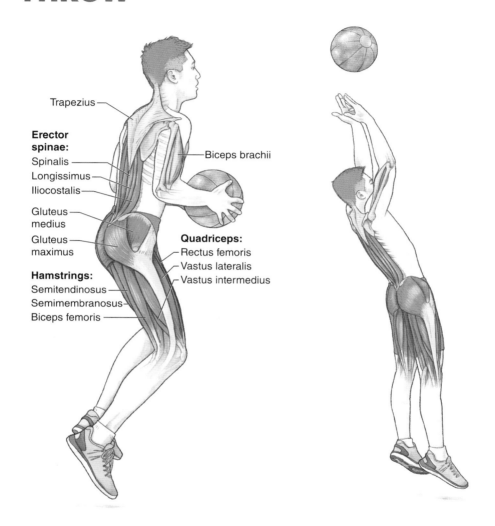

Trapezius

Erector spinae:
Spinalis
Longissimus
Iliocostalis

Gluteus medius
Gluteus maximus

Hamstrings:
Semitendinosus
Semimembranosus
Biceps femoris

Biceps brachii

Quadriceps:
Rectus femoris
Vastus lateralis
Vastus intermedius

Execution

1. Stand with feet approximately shoulder-width apart. Hold the medicine ball at chest height with both hands in preparation for an explosive reverse overhead throw. Face away from the direction of the throw.

2. Perform a countermovement to load the legs to prepare for a powerful jump. Jump forward, away from the direction of the throw, with a relatively powerful jump, keeping the ball at chest height.

3. After landing, descend into a squat and bring the ball to a position between the legs with the arms fully extended.

4. Initiate an explosive throw, driving from the lower body rapidly and pulling the ball along the length of the body.

5. Release the ball overhead with the posture of the body extended slightly backward to provide both height and distance to the throw.

Muscles Involved

Primary: Gluteus maximus, gluteus medius, quadriceps (rectus femoris, vastus lateralis, vastus intermedius, vastus medialis), hamstrings (biceps femoris, semitendinosus, semimembranosus), erector spinae (spinalis, longissimus, iliocostalis).

Secondary: Trapezius, biceps brachii.

Exercise Notes

A forward squat jump into a reverse overhead medicine-ball throw can enhance overall lower-body power as well as condition explosive changes of direction. The forward jump combined with the pulling motion of the reverse throw stimulates muscles of both the anterior and posterior. The loading of the lower body by the jumping motion stimulates greater muscle recruitment for the throwing motion. It is important to maintain proper posture throughout the exercise, particularly on the landing of the jump and preparation for the throw. Jump explosively as part of the throw, displacing your body backward.

VARIATION

Multiple Squat Jumps and Reverse Overhead Medicine-Ball Throw

Multiple squat jumps preceding a reverse overhead medicine-ball throw can combine elastic power with an explosive singular effort. The multiple jumps should be moderate in distance and effort. If you achieve too much forward momentum, it can be harder to reverse the direction of effort and complete an effective reverse overhead throw.

LATERAL SQUAT JUMP AND ROTATIONAL MEDICINE-BALL THROW

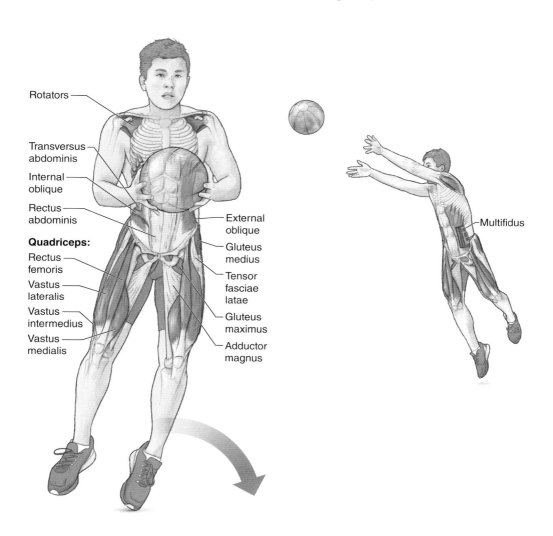

Rotators

Transversus abdominis

Internal oblique

Rectus abdominis

Quadriceps:

Rectus femoris

Vastus lateralis

Vastus intermedius

Vastus medialis

External oblique

Gluteus medius

Tensor fasciae latae

Gluteus maximus

Adductor magnus

Multifidus

Execution

1. Stand with feet approximately shoulder-width apart. Hold the medicine ball at waist height with both hands in preparation for an explosive rotational throw.

2. Start the exercise with a lateral jump of moderate distance. As the landing of the jump approaches, position the medicine ball to the outside hip in preparation for a strong rotational medicine-ball throw.

3. After landing the lateral jump, initiate a powerful medicine-ball throw across the body, turning the shoulders in the direction of the throw.

4. The force of the rotational throw should result in your body's following the direction of the throw upon release of the medicine ball.

Muscles Involved

Primary: Gluteus maximus, gluteus medius, quadriceps (rectus femoris, vastus lateralis, vastus intermedius, vastus medialis), transversus abdominis, internal oblique, external oblique, multifidus, rotators.

Secondary: Rectus abdominis, erector spinae (iliocostalis, longissimus, spinalis), tensor fasciae latae, adductor magnus, gluteus maximus.

Exercise Notes

The lateral jump into a rotational throw simulates a powerful change of direction because the rotation of the shoulders and torso typically precedes multidirectional movements. The exercise can begin with lateral jumps of shorter distances. As the training program progresses, larger lateral jumps can produce greater landing forces and more complete recruitment of lower-body muscles to contribute to a powerful rotational throw. You can perform throws on the same side or as alternate-side throws for each set.

VARIATION

Lateral Bound and Rotational Medicine-Ball Throw

As an alternative to a double-leg lateral jump, you can do a lateral bound from one leg to another before a rotational medicine-ball throw. The lateral bound can be quick and short, or it can be long and powerful. This variation provides an effective exercise for developing single-leg power for multidirectional movement.

MEDICINE-BALL PUSH THROW AND SPRINT

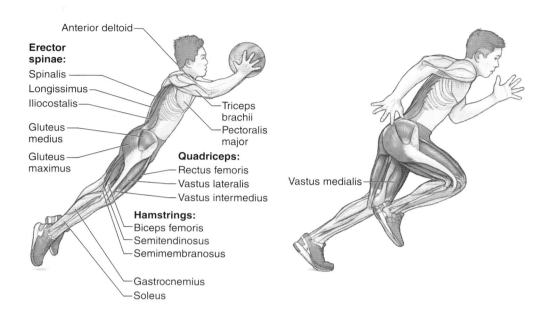

Anterior deltoid

Erector spinae:
Spinalis
Longissimus
Iliocostalis

Gluteus medius

Gluteus maximus

Triceps brachii

Pectoralis major

Quadriceps:
Rectus femoris
Vastus lateralis
Vastus intermedius

Hamstrings:
Biceps femoris
Semitendinosus
Semimembranosus

Gastrocnemius
Soleus

Vastus medialis

Execution

1. Stand with feet approximately hip-width apart. Hold the medicine ball at chest height with both hands in preparation for an explosive push throw.

2. Prepare for the medicine-ball throw by descending into a partial squat with the ball at chest height. Begin rolling forward onto the balls of the feet.

3. Initiate an explosive medicine-ball push throw with full-body extension from shoulders to ankles.

4. After release of the medicine ball, step into the first stride and initiate an arm drive, maintaining optimal acceleration posture.

5. Complete a sprint acceleration over 10 to 30 meters, maintaining efficient technique throughout the length of the run.

Muscles Involved

Primary: Gluteus maximus, gluteus medius, quadriceps (rectus femoris, vastus lateralis, vastus intermedius, vastus medialis), hamstrings (biceps femoris, semitendinosus, semimembranosus), erector spinae (spinalis, longissimus, iliocostalis).

Secondary: Pectoralis major, triceps brachii, anterior deltoid, soleus, gastrocnemius.

Exercise Notes

The medicine-ball push throw into a sprint is one of the most fundamental strength and acceleration exercises. The effort required for overcoming the inertia of both the body and the medicine ball will transfer to easier starting efforts for basic sprint training. As with any exercise, an effective starting position is key to ensuring powerful and efficient mechanics. You must keep the medicine ball on the chest at the start of the movement. The simultaneous application of force through both feet on the start of the push movement is required for getting both the body and the medicine ball moving quickly, setting the tone for a strong acceleration.

VARIATION

Medicine-Ball Push Throw and Sprint From Offset Stance

Using an offset stance on the medicine-ball push throw creates a more practical foot placement for many sports. The feet are slightly staggered so that the toes of the rear foot are parallel with the back heel of the front foot. Similar to the parallel stance, the initial application of force is through both feet. The rear foot separates from the ground first, with the front foot pushing longer to complete the starting movement. Foot placement for the offset stance should be hip-width apart with the toes of the rear foot lining up parallel to the heel of the front foot.

REVERSE OVERHEAD MEDICINE-BALL THROW AND SPRINT

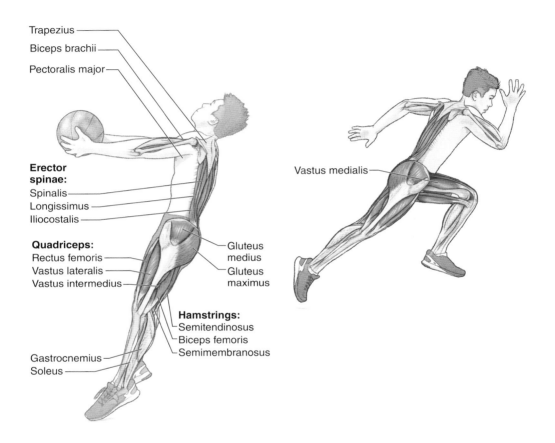

Trapezius

Biceps brachii

Pectoralis major

Erector spinae:
Spinalis
Longissimus
Iliocostalis

Quadriceps:
Rectus femoris
Vastus lateralis
Vastus intermedius

Gastrocnemius
Soleus

Gluteus medius
Gluteus maximus

Hamstrings:
Semitendinosus
Biceps femoris
Semimembranosus

Vastus medialis

Execution

1. Stand with feet approximately hip-width apart, facing away from the direction of the throw and sprint. Hold the medicine ball at waist height with arms extended in preparation for an explosive throw.

2. Descend into a squat with the ball lowering between the ankles. The torso should remain upright and the spine neutral throughout the squat.

3. Rapidly jump out of the squat, keeping the arms extended until you achieve full hip extension. Once you achieve full extension, the arms can finish pulling the ball overhead. Fully extend the body backward, driving the ball at an angle of 40 to 45 degrees.

4. After release of the medicine ball, turn the head and shoulders toward the direction of the sprint. As you conclude the 180-degree turn, begin pumping the arms and stepping into the first stride for the sprint start.

5. Complete a sprint acceleration over 10 to 30 meters, maintaining efficient technique throughout the length of the run.

Muscles Involved

Primary: Gluteus maximus, gluteus medius, quadriceps (rectus femoris, vastus lateralis, vastus intermedius, vastus medialis), hamstrings (biceps femoris, semitendinosus, semimembranosus), erector spinae (spinalis, longissimus, iliocostalis).

Secondary: Trapezius, biceps brachii, soleus, gastrocnemius.

Exercise Notes

The reverse overhead medicine-ball throw incorporates a powerful pulling motion into the start of this combination exercise. While a pushing throw uses more anterior muscles, pulling the medicine ball overhead uses more posterior muscles for propulsion of the ball. The rotation of the body into the sprint start also requires greater body control and agility before the acceleration.

VARIATION

Jump Into Reverse Overhead Medicine-Ball Throw and Sprint

The throw and sprint sequence can be preceded by a powerful jump forward to simulate an explosive change of direction in the opposite direction. The jump need not be maximal for the first few sessions. As you become more comfortable with the eccentric forces encountered in the jump-to-throw transition, you can incorporate a jump of greater length gradually through the progression.

ROTATIONAL MEDICINE-BALL THROW AND SPRINT

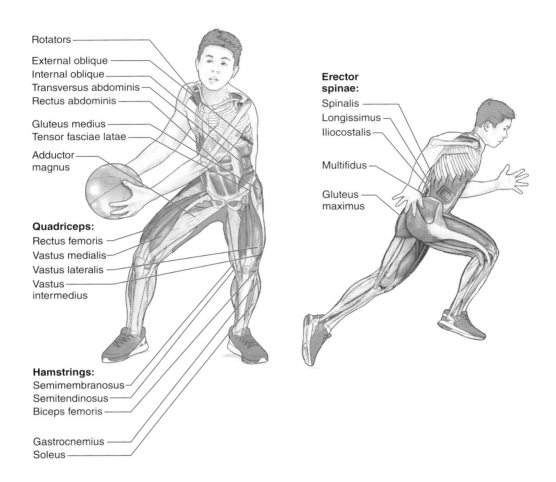

Rotators

External oblique
Internal oblique
Transversus abdominis
Rectus abdominis

Gluteus medius
Tensor fasciae latae

Adductor magnus

Quadriceps:
Rectus femoris
Vastus medialis
Vastus lateralis
Vastus intermedius

Hamstrings:
Semimembranosus
Semitendinosus
Biceps femoris

Gastrocnemius
Soleus

Erector spinae:
Spinalis
Longissimus
Iliocostalis

Multifidus

Gluteus maximus

Execution

1. Stand with feet approximately hip-width apart, facing perpendicular to the direction of the throw and sprint. Hold the medicine ball at waist height with arms extended in preparation for an explosive throw.

2. Take the ball to the far side of the body, away from the direction of the throw, to stretch the muscles of the core and upper extremities in preparation for a powerful rotational throw.

3. Explosively throw the ball across the body in the direction of the sprint, rapidly rotating the shoulders and torso 90 degrees.

4. The force of the throw will pull the body into the direction of the throw. As the body rotates forward, step into the first stride of the sprint, initiating a powerful arm drive to complete the running motion.

5. Complete a sprint acceleration over 10 to 30 meters, maintaining efficient technique throughout the length of the run.

Muscles Involved

Primary: Transversus abdominis, internal oblique, external oblique, multifidus, rotators, gluteus maximus, gluteus medius, quadriceps (rectus femoris, vastus lateralis, vastus intermedius, vastus medialis).

Secondary: Hamstrings (biceps femoris, semitendinosus, semimembranosus), erector spinae (spinalis, longissimus, iliocostalis), soleus, gastrocnemius, tensor fasciae latae, adductor magnus.

Exercise Notes

A rotational pass preceding a sprint effort simulates a powerful change of direction that is often required for sporting movements. Because upper-body rotational actions precede multidirectional movements, use of a medicine-ball throw can develop greater strength and power before explosive lower-body efforts. The upper-body rotational throw begins with strong lower-body involvement, pushing with the feet through the ground. The transfer of power from the ground through the core and out through the arms facilitates a quicker starting motion. Perform a high-velocity throw that transitions smoothly into a running motion without overextending through the throw.

VARIATION

Lateral Jump in Opposite Direction of Sprint

A powerful throw in the opposite direction of the sprint requires you to reverse the direction of momentum in the form of a sprint. The throw can be short and quick to simulate a quick change of direction, or it can be longer and more powerful to simulate a more profound deceleration before a sprint. In both cases, it is important to work on rotational throws on both sides of the body to prepare for all potential changes of direction in a sport.

CONSECUTIVE BROAD JUMPS INTO A SPRINT

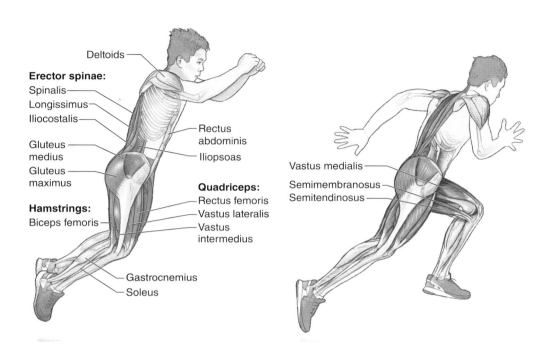

Deltoids

Erector spinae:
Spinalis
Longissimus
Iliocostalis

Gluteus medius
Gluteus maximus

Hamstrings:
Biceps femoris

Rectus abdominis
Iliopsoas

Quadriceps:
Rectus femoris
Vastus lateralis
Vastus intermedius

Gastrocnemius
Soleus

Vastus medialis
Semimembranosus
Semitendinosus

Execution

1. Start with the feet hip-width apart and moderate knee flexion. Before initiating the first broad jump, perform a moderate countermovement to create greater force production with the legs and strong hip extension. A strong double-arm swing accompanies the jump takeoff, driving the body powerfully forward and upward.

2. While it is important to emphasize horizontal distance in these jumps, it is also critical to achieve a takeoff trajectory of no lower than 30 degrees on each jump.

3. Land on both feet just slightly in front of your center of mass, allowing for the conservation of momentum and both vertical and horizontal force. The feet will land relatively flat, with the landing forces absorbed in the quadriceps, gluteal muscles, and the lower back.

4. Consecutive landings and takeoffs should involve moderate knee flexion: enough to safely absorb the landing forces and create propulsion for the next jump but not so much that you lose horizontal velocity and distance.

5. The transition from the final jump into the sprint should include a moderate torso lean forward to prepare for a sprint acceleration posture. Complete the acceleration over 10 to 30 meters, maintaining efficient technique throughout the length of the run.

Muscles Involved

Primary: Gluteus maximus, gluteus medius, quadriceps (rectus femoris, vastus lateralis, vastus intermedius, vastus medialis), hamstrings (biceps femoris, semitendinosus, semimembranosus), erector spinae (spinalis, longissimus, iliocostalis).

Secondary: Deltoids, rectus abdominis, iliopsoas, soleus, gastrocnemius.

Exercise Notes

Multiple explosive broad jumps (two to five jumps) before a sprint effort reinforce the powerful hip extension required for effective acceleration strides. The broad jumps should be maximal in effort but also performed in a manner that allows for successive jumps to achieve greater and greater acceleration before the sprint. Takeoffs and landings for these jumps must be quick and brief with minimal ground contacts to attain greater horizontal velocity. The arms are also maximally involved in driving upward and forward through the jumps. The final jump preceding the sprint should transition smoothly into the running motion, with the first stride touching down beneath the hips. The series of broad jumps will create adequate momentum to enter the sprint at a midacceleration velocity.

VARIATION

Lateral Broad Jumps Into a Sprint

Broad jumps with a lateral deviation before a sprint can simulate the forces experienced in a multidirectional sport movement. Vary the magnitude of lateral deviation on the broad jumps, depending on your sporting needs. A football running back may perform significant lateral jumps before a linear sprint, while a soccer player may implement shorter, quicker lateral jumps.

BOUNDING INTO A SPRINT

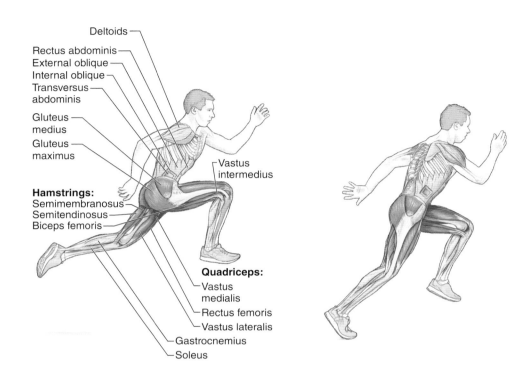

Deltoids
Rectus abdominis
External oblique
Internal oblique
Transversus abdominis
Gluteus medius
Gluteus maximus
Hamstrings:
Semimembranosus
Semitendinosus
Biceps femoris
Vastus intermedius
Quadriceps:
Vastus medialis
Rectus femoris
Vastus lateralis
Gastrocnemius
Soleus

Execution

1. Drive one knee forward, matching the effort with a single-arm drive with the opposite arm. The opposite leg extends powerfully in an elongated stride.

2. During the flight phase, the lead leg prepares for ground contact and begins a powerful downward sweep with the intent of landing midfoot. The opposite leg begins driving forward to pass the landing leg on ground contact and begins an upward and forward drive. Arms swing powerfully in opposition to counterbalance the action of the lower body.

3. Alternate the elongated strides in a rhythmic fashion over the length of the bounding set, driving for height and distance and maintaining short ground contact times on landing.

4. As the bounds progress over distance, increase the frequency of strides, producing a more rapid stride rate. The bounds gradually transition into sprint strides and a natural running motion.

5. The progression from bounds to sprint strides occurs over 10 to 30 meters, depending on the objective of the exercise. Ensure that the transition develops smoothly with no abrupt changes in posture, technique, or limb velocities.

Muscles Involved

Primary: Gluteus maximus, gluteus medius, quadriceps (rectus femoris, vastus lateralis, vastus intermedius, vastus medialis), hamstrings (biceps femoris, semitendinosus, semimembranosus).

Secondary: Transversus abdominis, internal oblique, external oblique, rectus abdominis, deltoids, soleus, gastrocnemius.

Exercise Notes

Transitioning from alternate-leg bounding to full-speed sprinting is a useful combination exercise for developing greater stride power and, ultimately, improved stride length. You will learn to appreciate the relationship between bounding and sprinting in the same drill, balancing stride length with stride frequency. Ensure that you blend the two exercises gradually over a suitable distance with no abrupt changes in any aspect of the movement.

VARIATION

Lateral Bounds Into a Sprint

Lateral bounds preceding a sprint provide an additional quality to the exercise. The lateral bounds can simulate the demands of the agility requirements of a specific sport. In this exercise, the transition between lateral bounds and the sprint can be gradual or it can be very abrupt, depending on the objectives of the exercise. If the exercise is intended to simulate a sport-specific scenario, a series of quick lateral bounds over 5 meters could be followed by an intense sprint over 10 meters. This drill could simulate the physical demands of a basketball athlete guarding on defense and then sprinting into a fast break.

LOW HURDLE JUMPS INTO A SPRINT

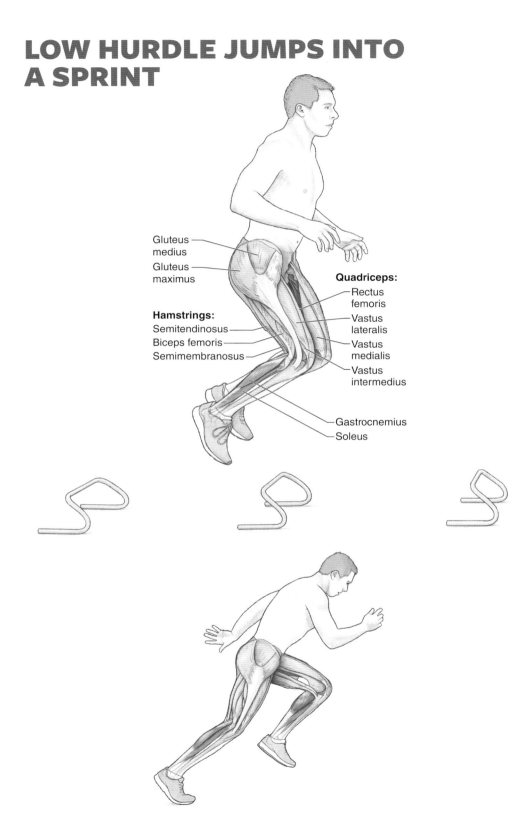

Gluteus medius

Gluteus maximus

Quadriceps:

Rectus femoris

Vastus lateralis

Vastus medialis

Vastus intermedius

Hamstrings:

Semitendinosus

Biceps femoris

Semimembranosus

Gastrocnemius

Soleus

Execution

1. Start the series of jumps with a tall posture and an emphasis on light and quick two-foot ground contacts between hurdles. Because the hurdles are low, emphasize active ground contacts to condition the muscles and tendons of the calves and feet. The point of contact on ground contact is the balls of the feet.

2. Travel over the hurdles in a quick but even rhythm with the arms swinging rapidly and over a relatively short range of motion, maintaining tall posture with the torso and head.

3. The horizontal speed of the exercise should be relatively quick with less energy devoted to achieving vertical height on each jump.

4. On the last hurdle, separate the feet and land with one leg to start the sprint sequence. The body should have a slight forward lean entering into the sprint.

5. Finish with a sprint acceleration over 10 to 30 meters, maintaining efficient technique throughout the length of the run.

Muscles Involved

Primary: Soleus, gastrocnemius.

Secondary: Gluteus maximus, gluteus medius, quadriceps (rectus femoris, vastus lateralis, vastus intermedius, vastus medialis), hamstrings (biceps femoris, semitendinosus, semimembranosus).

Exercise Notes

The use of quick jumps over low hurdles before a sprint prepares the lower legs for short and efficient ground contacts. The pistoning action of the legs during the hurdle jumps provides a good preparatory exercise immediately before the sprint effort. Hurdles should be relatively close together but with enough space to ensure safe ground contacts.

Groups of athletes can be positioned in two or three parallel lines to provide a competitive environment in which they race each other through the hurdles and sprints.

VARIATION

Multidirectional Low Hurdles Into a Sprint

A combination of low hurdles arranged to elicit forward and lateral jumps can be useful in preparing for quick, explosive multidirectional movements before a maximal sprint. Numerous combinations of jumps can be assembled. However, it is important to make sure that the number of jumps before a sprint is not excessive. The entire exercise, including the sprint, should not last more than 8 seconds, ensuring that speed qualities are being developed. Take adequate rest breaks between sets.

HIGH HURDLE JUMPS INTO A SPRINT

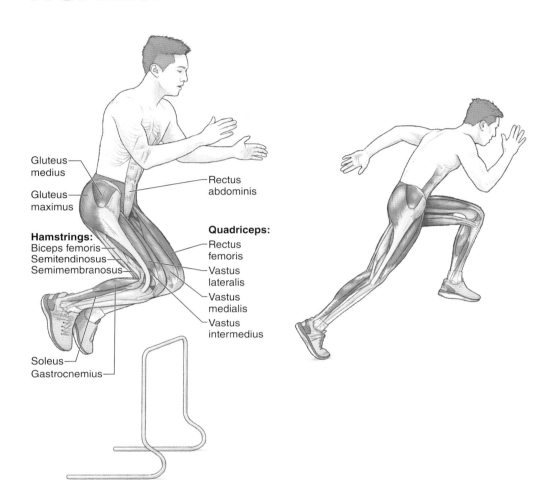

Gluteus medius

Gluteus maximus

Rectus abdominis

Hamstrings:
Biceps femoris
Semitendinosus
Semimembranosus

Quadriceps:
Rectus femoris

Vastus lateralis

Vastus medialis

Vastus intermedius

Soleus
Gastrocnemius

Execution

1. High hurdle jumps require a more significant effort during takeoff, flight, and landing. The takeoff must be maximal in effort. Extend powerfully at the hip to attain the appropriate height for flight over the hurdle. The arms swing powerfully upward to assist in the effort.

2. Flight over the hurdle includes lifting the knees, similar to a tuck jump, to ensure adequate clearance over the barrier.

3. To prepare to land, dorsiflex the feet to ensure a stiff and elastic landing on the balls of the feet. A quick and powerful elastic landing will ensure maximum height on successive jumps.

4. When landing over the last high hurdle, move into a split stance that sets you up for a sprint start.

5. Finish with a sprint acceleration over 10 to 30 meters, maintaining efficient technique throughout the length of the run.

Muscles Involved

Primary: Gluteus maximus, gluteus medius, quadriceps (rectus femoris, vastus lateralis, vastus intermedius, vastus medialis), soleus, gastrocnemius.

Secondary: Rectus abdominis, iliopsoas, hamstrings (biceps femoris, semitendinosus, semimembranosus).

Exercise Notes

High hurdle jumps before a sprint develop maximal force production qualities in the legs. Although the ground contact times for high hurdle jumps may be longer than those in sprinting, the maximal recruitment characteristics of such explosive jumps will carry over to other aspects of sport performance including change of direction and deceleration. While a regular hurdle jump routine may include up to 10 hurdles per set, using 5 hurdles or fewer before a sprint would be appropriate for this combination exercise.

VARIATION

High Hurdle Jumps Into a Sprint With Weighted Vest or Belt

The addition of a relatively small load to the body can build explosive qualities through jumps and sprints. The load can be 5 to 10 extra pounds on a vest or a belt. Although this may seem like a very small load, when combined with maximal jumps and sprints, the load is magnified several times over. The load provides an extra stimulus for the vertical component of both the jumps and sprints. After two or three sets of loaded jumps and sprints, you can take off the vest or belt. You will feel exceptionally lighter and more explosive for the remaining sets.

LATERAL HURDLE JUMP A INTO SPRINT

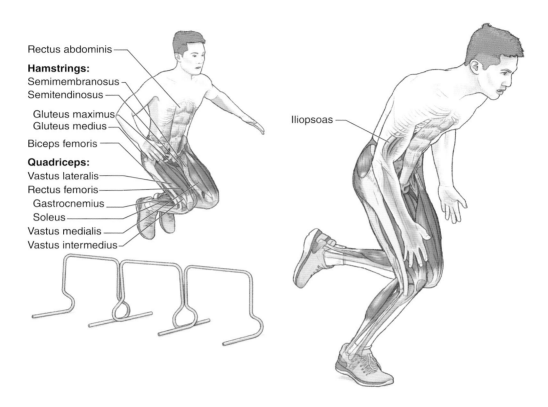

Rectus abdominis

Hamstrings:
Semimembranosus
Semitendinosus

Gluteus maximus
Gluteus medius

Biceps femoris

Quadriceps:
Vastus lateralis
Rectus femoris
Gastrocnemius
Soleus
Vastus medialis
Vastus intermedius

Iliopsoas

Execution

1. Arrange a series of hurdles in a line positioned end to end. Begin by jumping laterally and slightly forward over the first hurdle.

2. Jump in a zigzag pattern back and forth over the hurdles. Depending on the height of the hurdles, you may need significant hip flexion and knee lift at the top of each jump.

3. Ground contacts for each landing will be short and quick, taking advantage of the elastic response in the feet and lower legs. The arms assist in the execution of each jump, driving forward and up in a rhythmic fashion.

4. At the end of the line of hurdles or after a specific number of jumps, perform a linear sprint over 10 to 30 meters.

Muscles Involved

Primary: Gluteus maximus, gluteus medius, quadriceps (rectus femoris, vastus lateralis, vastus intermedius, vastus medialis), soleus, gastrocnemius.

Secondary: Rectus abdominis, iliopsoas, hamstrings (biceps femoris, semi-tendinosus, semimembranosus).

Exercise Notes

You can perform the lateral hurdle jumps over low or high hurdles depending on the objectives of the exercise and your abilities. Lower hurdles allow you to focus on tall posture and quick ground contacts. Higher hurdles require greater attention to hip flexion and jump height while also ensuring elastic ground contacts. In both cases, the exercise finishes with a fast sprint over 10 to 30 meters. Perform one to six lateral jumps before the sprint. The intent is to condition you to perform quick and explosive lateral movements before a sprint burst, very similar to what regularly occurs in numerous sports.

VARIATION

Lateral Single-Leg Hurdle Jumps Into a Sprint

Using a series of low hurdles arranged in a line, perform lateral jumps back and forth across the barriers with a single leg before a sprint. Because of the significant demands placed on a single leg, you should perform fewer jump repetitions. It is common to perform no more than five jumps at most before a sprint. This exercise significantly strengthens the muscles of the lower legs and feet, building explosive qualities for movements that require power and agility.

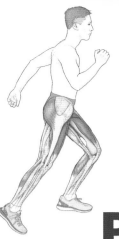

9

INJURY PREVENTION AND REHABILITATION

I njury prevention and rehabilitation have long been linked in the sports medicine world and, in fact, have many similarities. When preparing for sport performance, the first rule is to do no harm. Plyometrics for injury prevention and rehabilitation consist of exercises of various speeds, intensities, heights, and directions. Before implementing a program, you must consider several other factors including age, developmental level, injury history, training history, and sport. In addition, basic levels of strength and motor control are required for more advanced exercises.

From an athletic standpoint, injury prevention involves the development of numerous physical qualities including mobility, stability, work capacity, strength, power, speed, and endurance. A basic understanding of the scientific principles of biology, anatomy, physiology, kinesiology, biomechanics, and sport are required for injury-prevention programming. Rehabilitation from athletic injury involves a further understanding of the biology of injury and healing, surgical interventions, and rehabilitation principles. The goals for both injury prevention and rehabilitation remain the same: to prepare you to meet and sustain the physical demands of your chosen sport.

Much of the focus of plyometrics for injury prevention and rehabilitation centers on assessment of risk of injury. Plyometrics provides an excellent means for identifying risk in healthy populations and identifying limiting factors in return to play for injured athletes. This chapter provides you with a basic understanding of plyometric injury risk assessments and progressions for injury rehabilitation.

INJURY PREVENTION

Plyometric training has been shown to be an effective tool in correcting neuromuscular deficits and preventing injuries (Chu and Cordier 2000). As an athlete, you must learn and consistently demonstrate proper starts, stops, runs, cuts, jumps, landings, and control of your body during skill movements. Plyometric exercises for injury prevention must be progressive and provide the proper stress to improve your ability to control your trunk and develop core stability, movement skills, strength, and power to achieve success in sport.

A great deal of research regarding the use of plyometric training for injury prevention has been directed toward reducing anterior cruciate ligament (ACL) injuries. Multiple studies have shown that plyometric neuromuscular programs may significantly reduce the risk of ACL injuries in females (Hewett et al. 1999; Hewett, Myer, and Ford 2006; Hewett, Di Stasi, and Myer 2013; Ladenhauf, Graziano, and Marx 2013). In addition, several studies support the finding that this type of training improves athletic performance (Hewett, Di Stasi, and Myer 2013; Myer et al. 2005). ACL prevention programs focus on jumping, hopping, bounding, landing, starting, and stopping exercises performed with proper technique and motor control. Through plyometrics, you learn to stabilize and control your center of mass over your base of support in all planes of movement, thereby reducing stress on the lower body.

If you are prone to injury, you can use plyometric exercises for assessing faulty movement patterns, muscle imbalances, strength deficits, core control, and other deficiencies that may predispose you to further injury. A plyometric assessment provides the framework for building a neuromuscular and plyometric injury-prevention program. Researchers have identified four neuromuscular imbalances associated with the underlying ACL injury mechanisms: ligament dominant, quadriceps dominant, leg dominant, and trunk dominant (Hewett et al. 2010).

Ligament-dominant athletes tend to control movement by hanging on their ligaments instead of using the muscular system to stabilize their bodies. Upon landing, their hips and knees collapse inward in a knock-kneed fashion. These athletes cannot adequately control their hips, forcing the ligaments—not the primary movers (glutes, quadriceps, hamstrings, and calves)—to control motion creating increased stress at the hip, knee, and ankle joints. If you do not have the ability to activate the trunk and hip stabilizers, they create high forces that cause the knees to come together.

Quadriceps-dominant athletes rely on their quadriceps muscles to provide strength and stability at the knee joint. The quadriceps provides strength and stability only at the front of the knee, thereby limiting the ability to control motion in all three planes of movement. Upon landing from drops or jumps, these athletes may display a wobble motion about the knee joint. Athletes who land with minimal knee bend and flat feet may also be identified as quadriceps dominant. The gluteal muscles control the position of the femur in all three planes of movement, so developing strength and stability in the posterior chain becomes crucial for these athletes.

Leg-dominant athletes display an imbalance in the strength, coordination, and control between the right and left legs. In effect, one leg or muscle becomes more dominant, upsetting the natural balance of the biomechanical system. Muscle imbalances and strength asymmetries affect overall stability, increasing risk of injury.

Trunk-dominant athletes have difficulty controlling their trunks and the coordination of their core musculature. When this occurs in jumping and landing activities, you get a large ground reaction force that cannot be dissipated due to the excessive motion of the trunk, creating increased force and torque to the ligaments of the knee.

Unlike the lower extremities, there is limited research for upper-body plyometric training regarding injury prevention and injury rehabilitation. Only recently has there been advancement in this area. In theory, plyometric training provides the stimulus for achieving all of the necessary components of trunk and shoulder health and function. The majority of upper-body plyometric exercises are performed through the use of medicine balls or similar objects. When performed properly exercises using these implements provide the necessary force from the ground through the kinetic chain, developing strength and power while assisting in functional skill development. Plyometric training also provides necessary eccentric strength for controlling joint motion, which is essential for injury prevention.

Plyometric training for injury prevention of the upper body follows the same principles. You must have a baseline of upper-extremity strength and motor control before participation. Exercises must be progressive and provide the proper stress to improve your ability to control the trunk and develop core stability and power to achieve success.

For the shoulders to function well, they must have adequate scapular stability, rotator cuff range of motion and strength, and thoracic mobility. (See figure 9.1 for the muscles of the scapula and rotator cuff.) The scapula provides a stable base for the arm to function. The muscles that stabilize the scapula (trapezius, rhomboids, serratus anterior, levator scapulae, latissimus dorsi) must be able to

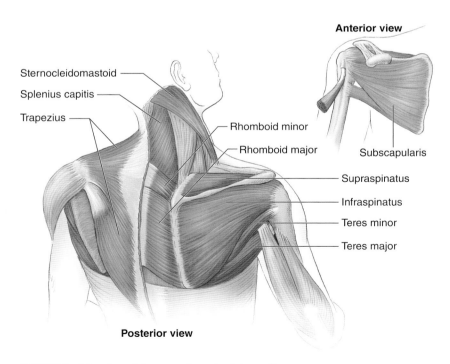

FIGURE 9.1   Muscles of the scapula and rotator cuff.

control motion to allow for greater strength and power of the arm. The main purpose of the rotator cuff musculature (supraspinatus, infraspinatus, subscapularis, teres minor) is to maintain the humeral head in the glenoid fossa. A strong rotator cuff allows for proper mechanics of the glenohumeral joint by maintaining proper positioning and control of the humerus within the joint. A mobile thoracic spine allows both the scapular stabilizers and rotator cuff muscles to function more efficiently in controlling scapulohumeral rhythm and neuromuscular timing without compensation.

INJURY REHABILITATION

There is a fine line between tissue healing and rehabilitation. Injured joints and soft-tissue structures are compromised and do not tolerate exercise volumes and intensities as normal tissue does. Be careful not to negatively stress the healing environment in a rehabilitation setting. You need to develop a strategy that allows for successful return and sustenance of competition. Before participation, you must first develop functional stability and concentric, isometric, and eccentric strength to build the foundation and decrease the chances of reinjury.

You have many exercises and progressions to choose from when incorporating plyometrics into a rehabilitation program. For this reason, you need to keep things basic. Training volume, intensity, frequency, and recovery must be closely monitored in a rehabilitation setting. In effect, every exercise and training session becomes an assessment for warning signs such as pain, swelling, and fatigue. You must be able to continually demonstrate good technique and motor control with simple body-weight exercises before more advanced exercises and loads. To reduce warning signs, simple rules for progressions are to move from easy to hard, simple to complex, and slow to fast types of plyometric exercises. You must develop adequate ability in performing bilateral extremity and noninjured single-extremity types of plyometric exercises before initiating injured-extremity exercises. No rehabilitation program is written in stone, either; you must be willing to adapt to your current physical and mental state and progress or regress plyometric activity accordingly.

You may use plyometric assessments created for determining return-to-play status; however, plyometric assessments are just one of many factors involved when returning to play, and you must use these assessments in conjunction with other performance-related testing.

INJURY PREVENTION AND REHABILITATION ASSESSMENTS

Plyometric assessments provide valuable information regarding movement, strength, power, stability, and muscle imbalances and asymmetries. These assessments are the framework for building a plyometric program. Many of the exercises described in previous chapters, such as depth drops and squat jumps, may be used for both injury prevention and rehabilitation after completion of assessment.

For lower-body assessments, you may be at increased risk of injury if you display one or more of the following deficiencies:

Ligament Dominance
- Knock-kneed landing or inward collapse of landing knee
- Knee moving past the toe
- Narrow foot landing

Quadriceps Dominance
- Stiff-leg landing
- Excessive noise on landing

Trunk Dominance
- Landing off balance
- Inability to maintain balance over base of support
- Thighs not reaching parallel at peak height
- Not landing in the same footprint as takeoff

Leg Dominance
- Favoring or hopping farther on one leg
- Legs unequal side to side during flight
- Unparallel foot placement

PLYOMETRIC PROGRESSIONS FOR INJURY REHABILITATION

When you are injured, one of the easiest ways to reintroduce plyometrics is through aquatic (pool) training. Pool training is an excellent choice because the buoyancy and hydrostatic pressure of the water reduce body weight and increase venous return, leading to improved circulation and decreased swelling and pain. You can work longer and safer in the water while increasing range of motion and aerobic strength and capacity. To reduce the chances of infection, surgical incisions must be well healed before initiating plyometrics in the water. As a general rule, begin in chest-deep water at submaximal intensities. Submaximal efforts will restrengthen muscles, tendons, and ligaments while reintroducing proper athletic patterning. Efforts may be repeated often as long as there are no signs or symptoms of pain and inflammation. However, a good rule is to allow 24 to 48 hours between sessions for adequate recovery. As you improve, the depth of the water may be reduced to waist level before opting for dryland training.

Progression for Basic Plyometric Pool Rehabilitation
1. Stationary jumps in place: Work up to 2 or 3 sets of 30 repetitions
2. Linear line jumps in place: Work up to 2 or 3 sets of 30 repetitions

3. Lateral line jumps in place: Work up to 2 or 3 sets of 30 repetitions

4. Linear jumps over distance: Work up to 2 or 3 sets of 20 repetitions

5. Lateral jumps over distance: Work up to 2 or 3 sets of 20 repetitions

6. Stationary skips in place: Work up to 2 or 3 sets of 30 repetitions

7. Linear skips over distance: Work up to 2 or 3 sets of 20 repetitions

8. Lateral skips over distance: Work up to 2 or 3 sets of 20 repetitions

9. Stationary hops in place: Work up to 2 or 3 sets of 30 repetitions

10. Linear hops in place: Work up to 2 or 3 sets of 30 repetitions

11. Lateral hops in place: Work up to 2 or 3 sets of 30 repetitions

12. Linear hops over distance: Work up to 2 or 3 sets of 20 repetitions

13. Lateral hops over distance: Work up to 2 or 3 sets of 20 repetitions

14. Linear bounds: Work up to 2 or 3 sets of 10 repetitions

15. Lateral bounds: Work up to 2 or 3 sets of 10 repetitions

16. Diagonal bounds: Work up to 2 or 3 sets of 10 repetitions

Exercises are completed at submaximal levels without pain or fatigue for the designated number of sets and repetitions before moving to the next progression. Closely monitor for pain and swelling during and after each session. The term *work up* refers to the number of repetitions per set. The goal is to complete the designated number of repetitions without stopping. However, you may need to work up to the number with frequent stops until you achieve the goal.

PROGRESSION FOR BASIC DRYLAND JUMP AND HOP PLYOMETRIC REHABILITATION

Submaximal intensities continue to be stressed once dryland training is initiated. Initially, perform exercises on mats or some type of softer surface to reduce compression and shearing forces on joints. The first three exercises in the progression are at low intensities; exercises 4 through 7 are at medium intensities; exercises 8 through 11 are at higher intensities. In general, training frequency starts at two days per week. Sets and repetitions depend on the exercise and your current state of healing. You must use good judgment so as not to create an inflammatory response. As you respond to the new training stresses, you may incorporate harder surfaces and higher volumes and intensities to build more strength, power, motor control, and endurance. As you progress, always be aware of training volume; increased volume with inadequate recovery produces fatigue, which may negatively affect muscles, tendons, and joints. Once maximum efforts are within reach, plyometric intensities increase while volumes decrease. Recovery may take up to 72 hours to ensure adequate recovery of soft tissues and central nervous system. The key is to progress in a linear fashion in order to maintain the fine line between tissue healing and rehabilitation.

From a rehabilitation standpoint, first you should complete the jump progression with proficiency, then complete the same exercises substituting jumps with hops on the noninjured side before completing them on the injured side. You may progress these exercises with the use of bands, increased hurdle and box heights, and multiple repetitions.

1. Leg-press jumps or hops: 2 or 3 sets of 6 to 8 repetitions
2. Linear jump or hop and stick: 2 or 3 sets of 6 to 8 repetitions
3. Submaximal linear jump or hop over distance: 2 or 3 sets of 8 to 10 repetitions
4. Hurdle jump or hop and stick (6-inch hurdle): 2 or 3 sets of 3 to 5 hurdles
5. Hurdle jump or hop with bounce (6-inch hurdle): 2 or 3 sets of 3 to 5 hurdles
6. Continuous hurdle jump or hop (6-inch hurdle): 2 or 3 sets of 3 to 5 hurdles
7. Static start box jump (9- to 12-inch box) or box hop (6- to 9-inch box): 2 or 3 sets of 3 or 4 repetitions
8. Squat jump or hop and stick: 2 or 3 sets of 3 or 4 repetitions
9. Broad jump or hop and stick: 2 or 3 sets of 2 or 3 repetitions
10. Depth drop (12- to 18-inch box): 2 or 3 sets of 2 or 3 repetitions
11. Depth drop to jump (12- to 18-inch box): 2 or 3 sets of 2 or 3 repetitions

PROGRESSION FOR BASIC SINGLE-ARM UPPER-BODY PLYOMETRIC REHABILITATION

Plyometric training for the upper extremities should begin with submaximal intensities. Rehabilitation parameters depend on your current state of healing, but training generally begins with a frequency of two days per week. The types of exercises move from isolated to functional. Initiate medicine-ball exercises with very light loads so volume follows a standard format of 2 or 3 sets of 10 repetitions.

1. Prone 90/90 external rotation catch
2. Half-kneeling 90/90 rhythmic medicine-ball wall toss
3. Half-kneeling 90/90 medicine-ball external rotation throw
4. Half-kneeling 90/90 reverse catch
5. Half-kneeling 90/90 reverse catch with rotation

As you respond to the new training stresses, you may incorporate higher volumes and intensities to build strength, power, motor control, and endurance. As with the lower extremities, the key is to progress in a linear fashion to maintain the fine line between tissue healing and rehabilitation.

REFERENCES

Abbott, B.C., and Aubert, X.M. 1952. The force exerted by active striated muscle during and after change of length. *Journal of Physiology,* 117: 77-86.

Bompa, T.O. 1993. *Power training for sport: Plyometrics for maximum power development.* Oakville, ON: Mosaic Press.

Bosco, C., and Komi, P.V. 1979. Mechanical characteristics and fiber composition of human leg extensor muscles. *European Journal of Applied Physiology* 41: 275-284.

Cavagna, G.A. 1977. Storage and utilization of elastic energy in skeletal muscle. *Exercise and Sport Science Review,* 5: 89-129.

Chu, D.A. 1984. Jumping into plyometrics. *NSCA Journal,* 6(6):51.

Chu, D.A., and Cordier, D.J. 2000. Plyometrics in rehabilitation. In *Knee ligament rehabilitation,* edited by T.S. Ellenbecker. New York, NY: Churchill Livingstone.

Chu, D.A. and Myer, G.D. 2013. *Plyometrics.* Champaign, IL: Human Kinetics.

Comyns, T.M., Harrison, A.J., and Hennessy, L.K. 2011. An investigation into the recovery process of a maximum stretch-shortening cycle fatigue protocol on drop and rebound jumps. *Journal of Strength and Conditioning Research,* 25(8): 2177-2184.

De Villarreal, E.S., Requena, B., and Newton, R.U. 2010. Does plyometric training improve strength performance? A meta-analysis. *Journal of Science and Medicine in Sport,* 13: 513-522.

Ebben, W.P., Carroll, R.M., and Simenz, C.J. 2004. Strength and conditioning practices of National Hockey League strength and conditioning coaches. *Journal of Strength and Conditioning Research,* 18: 889–897.

Ebben, W.P., Hintz, M.J., and Simenz, C.J. 2005. Strength and conditioning practices of Major League Baseball strength and conditioning coaches. *Journal of Strength and Conditioning Research,* 19: 538–546.

Enoka, R. 1997. Neural adaptations with chronic physical activity. *Journal of Biomechanics,* 30(5): 447-455.

Fukutani, A., Kurihara, T., and Isaka, T. 2015. Factors of force potentiation induced by stretch-shortening cycle in plantarflexors. *PLoS ONE,* 10(6): e0120579.

Herzog, W., and Leonard, T.R. 2000. The history dependence of force production in mammalian skeletal muscle following stretch-shortening and shortening-stretch cycles. *Journal of Biomechanics,* 33: 531-542.

Hewett, T.E., Di Stasi, S.L, and Myer, G.D. 2013. Current concepts for injury prevention in athletes after anterior cruciate ligament reconstruction. *American Journal of Sports Medicine* 41(1): 216–224.

Hewett, T.E., Ford, K.R., Hoogenboom, B.J., and Myer, G.D. 2010. Understanding and preventing ACL injuries: Current biomechanical and epidemiologic considerations—update 2010. *North American Journal of Sports Physical Therapy* 5(4): 234–251.

Hewett, T.E., Lindenfeld, T.N., Riccobene, J.V., and Noyes, F.N. 1999. The effect of neuromuscular training on the incidence of knee injury in female athletes: A prospective study. *American Journal of Sports Medicine* 27(6): 699–706.

Hewett, T.E., Myer, G.D., and Ford, K.R. 2006. Anterior cruciate ligament injuries in female athletes. Part I: Mechanisms and risk factors. *American Journal of Sports Medicine* 34(2): 299–311.

Hill, A.V. 1950. The series elastic component of muscle. *Royal Proceedings of the Royal Society of London*. Series B (137): 273-280.

Holcomb, W.R., Kleiner, D.M., and Chu, D.A. 1998. Plyometrics: Considerations for safe and effective training. *NSCA Journal of Strength and Conditioning*, 20(3): 36-41.

Komi, P.V. 1984. Physiological and biomechanical correlates of muscle function: Effects of muscle structure and stretch-shortening cycle on force and speed. *Exercise and Sports Sciences Reviews/ACSM*, 12: 81-121.

Komi, P.V. 2000. Stretch-shortening cycle: A powerful model to study normal and fatigued muscle. *Journal of Biomechanics*, 33(10): 1197-1206.

Ladenhauf, H.N., Graziano, J., and Marx, R.G. 2013. Anterior cruciate ligament prevention strategies: Are they effective in young athletes? Current concepts and review of literature. *Current Opinion in Pediatrics* 25(1): 64–71.

Myer, G.D., Ford, K.R., Palumbo, J.P., and Hewett, T.E. 2005. Neuromuscular training improves performance and lower-extremity biomechanics in female athletes. *Journal of Strength and Conditioning Research* 19(1): 51–60.

Nardone, M., and Schieppati, M. 1988. Shift of activity from slow to fast muscle during voluntary lengthening contractions of the triceps surae muscles in humans. *Journal of Physiology*, 395: 363-381.

Radcliffe, J.C., and Farentinos, R.C. 1985. *Plyometrics: Explosive power training* (2nd edition). Champaign, IL: Human Kinetics.

Rassier, D.E., Herzog, W., Wakeling, J., and Syme, D.A. 2003. Stretch-induced steady state force enhancement in single skeletal muscle fibers exceeds the isometric force at optimum fiber lengths. *Journal of Biomechanics*, 36: 1309-1316.

Saunders, P.U., Telford, R.D., and Pyne, D.B. 2006. Short-term plyometric training improves running economy in highly trained middle and long distance runners. *Journal of Strength and Conditioning Research*, November, 20(4): 947-954.

Simenz, C.J., Dugan, C.A., and Ebben, W.P. 2005. Strength and conditioning practices of National Basketball Association strength and conditioning coaches. *Journal of Strength and Conditioning Research*, 19: 495–504.

Spudich, J.A. 2001. The myosin swinging cross-bridge model. *Nature Reviews Molecular Cell Biology*, 2(5): 387-392.

Spurrs, R.W., Murphy, A.J., and Watsford, M.L. 2003. The effect of plyometric training on distance running performance. *European Journal of Applied Physiology* 89(1): 1-7.

Verkhoshansky, Y. 1969. Perspectives in the improvement of speed-strength preparation in jumpers. *Yessis Review of Soviet Physical Education and Sports*, 4(2): 28-29.

Verkhoshansky, Y. 1973. Depth jumping in the training of jumpers. *Track Technique*, 41: 1618-1619.

Wilson, G.J., Elliott, B.C., and Wood, G.A. 1991. The effect on performance of imposing a delay during a stretch-shorten cycle movement. *Journal of Medicine and Science in Sport and Exercise*, 23(3): 364-370.

Wilt, F. 1975. Plyometrics: What is it now and how it works. *Athletic Journal*, 55(5):76, 89-90.

EXERCISE FINDER

FOUNDATIONAL EXERCISES

BILATERAL LOWER-BODY EXERCISES

UPPER-BODY EXERCISES

CORE EXERCISES

COMBINATION PLYOMETRIC EXERCISES

ABOUT THE AUTHORS

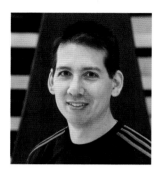

Derek Hansen, MASc, CSCS, has worked with athletes in speed, strength, and power sports since 1988. Originally a coach for track and field athletes, Hansen expanded his services to assist athletes in all sports, with an emphasis on speed development. As a coach and a consultant, he has worked with some of the top performers in the world, including Olympic medalists, world record holders, Canadian National team athletes, professional sports organizations and professional athletes from numerous sports. He has developed some of the top sprinters in British Columbia, and he continues to work with some of the fastest athletes in various sports.

Hansen has also served as a sport performance consultant or rehabilitation specialist to sports teams in the National Football League (NFL), National Basketball Association (NBA), National Hockey League (NHL), Major League Baseball (MLB), Major League Soccer (MLS), and National Collegiate Athletic Association (NCAA) Division I. From 2003 to 2016, he was the head strength and conditioning coach at Simon Fraser University. In each position, he has provided recommendations on how and when to use plyometric training for off-season preparation, in-season strength maintenance, and return-to-competition protocols following injury.

Steve Kennelly, MEd, ATC, CSCS, has been a member of the New York Football Giants medical team for more than 25 seasons and currently serves as their assistant head athletic trainer. Recognized as a leader in his field, Kennelly received the NFL Assistant Athletic Trainer of the Year Award for the National Football Conference (NFC) in 2012. In 1999 he was part of the Giants staff that was named the NFL Athletic Training Staff of the Year.

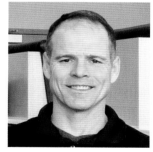

Both a certified athletic trainer and certified strength and conditioning specialist, Kennelly has served in various roles and medical committees for the National Football League, Professional Football Athletic Trainers' Society, National Athletic Trainers' Association, and the Athletic Trainers' Society of New Jersey. In 2013, after recognizing a need for quality instruction and programs in injury prevention, athletic development, postinjury reconditioning, and physical preparation, he founded Kennelly Athletics and Sports Medicine, LLC. His goal is to educate athletes, coaches, and parents on proper technique and progressions from fundamental movement patterns to advanced skills.